CHARLIE WATSON

COOK
EAT
RUN

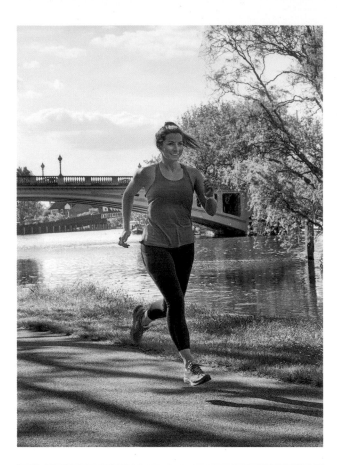

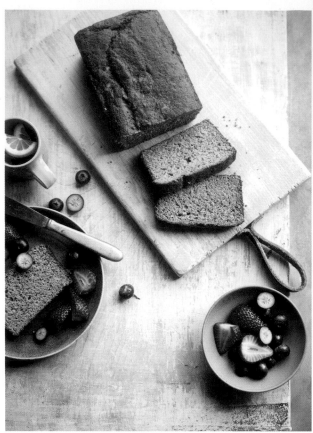

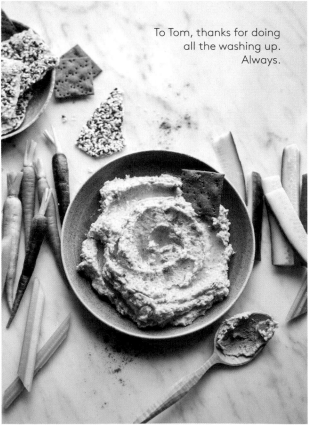

To Tom, thanks for doing
all the washing up.
Always.

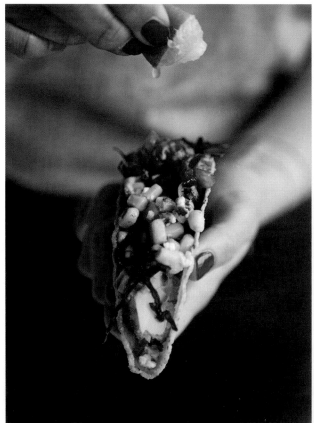

CHARLIE WATSON

COOK
EAT
RUN

Cook fast, boost performance with
over 75 ultimate recipes for runners

Photography by Maja Smend

Hardie Grant

QUADRILLE

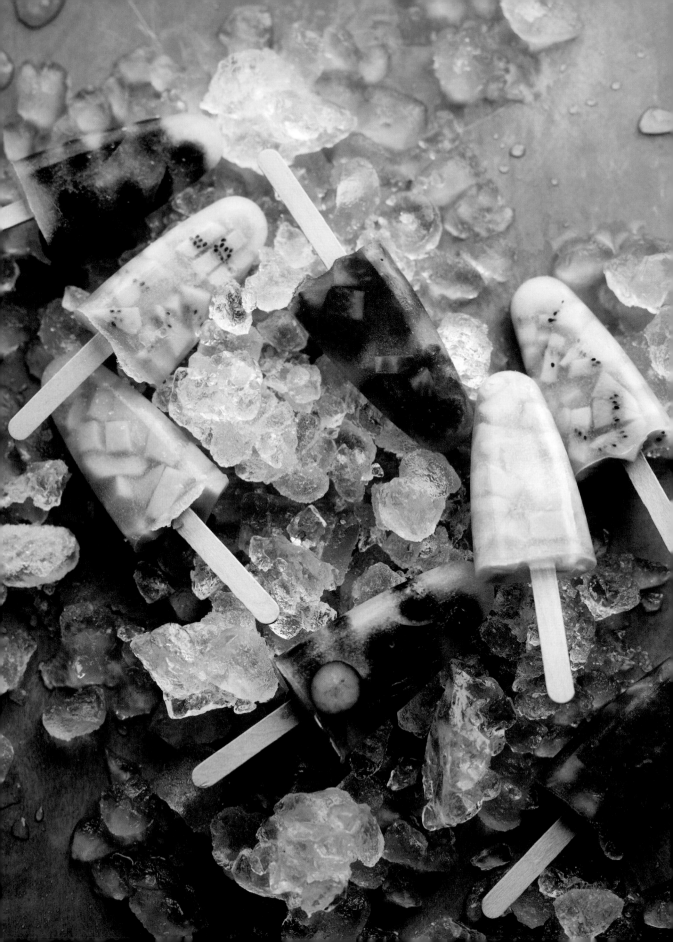

Contents

Introduction

I wrote this book after being inspired by Shalane Flanagan and Elyse Kopecky's book *Run Fast, Cook Fast, Eat Slow*. I loved their recipes and the concept behind the book, and wanted to create my own version that included speedy suppers, on-the-run fuel and post-workout meals, as well as baked goods. I wanted to put into action the recipe-writing skills taught to me by my friend and mentor Meike Beck at *Good Housekeeping* magazine, and combine them with the knowledge gained during my four-year dietetics degree, and share it in a simple, easy-to-digest format (metaphorically and physically speaking).

Nutrition can get so overcomplicated, with specialist ingredients and confusing, often seemingly contradictory, science. This book is aimed at runners of all levels – even those who are struggling to call themselves runners right now (side note: if you run, you're a runner, no matter your pace or distance). Whether you're building up for your first 5K, have decided to run a marathon, or are training for any length in-between (or beyond), I hope this book inspires you to get into the kitchen and rethink your nutrition, and encourages you to keep working towards your goals.

I started running because of grief. Losing one of my best friends, Vic, to depression at the end of our university days was my first experience of loss and I took it hard. Ten years ago, talking about mental health issues, or just 'not being OK', was more taboo. I wanted to do something positive in memory of him, to honour his life and, importantly, to raise funds and awareness for those struggling with their own mental health. So, I signed up for the 2011 London Marathon, with no real clue about how far a marathon was.

After being accepted onto the MIND team, I exaggerated and said I had already started training. That evening I went for my first run and made it just 100 metres down the street before having to stop and pretend to stretch. I was embarrassed to be so out of breath in front of the teens standing at the bus stop nearby.

Undeterred, I soon discovered running blogs, found a Hal Higdon beginner marathon training plan, and started to lace up my trainers three or four times per week. Unfortunately, my inexperience meant that I didn't stretch, strength- or cross-train, and so I found myself injured just a few weeks before the marathon that year. Luckily, I was able to defer my place and trained with renewed confidence, fitness and enthusiasm for the next year.

I finished my first marathon, the 2012 London Marathon, in 4 hours 54 minutes and 59 seconds. I didn't fuel during that first race – no gels, just a couple of sweets grabbed from course spectators. But there was no 'never again' moment after crossing that finish line. I knew immediately that not only did I want to do it again, but next time I wanted to run faster.

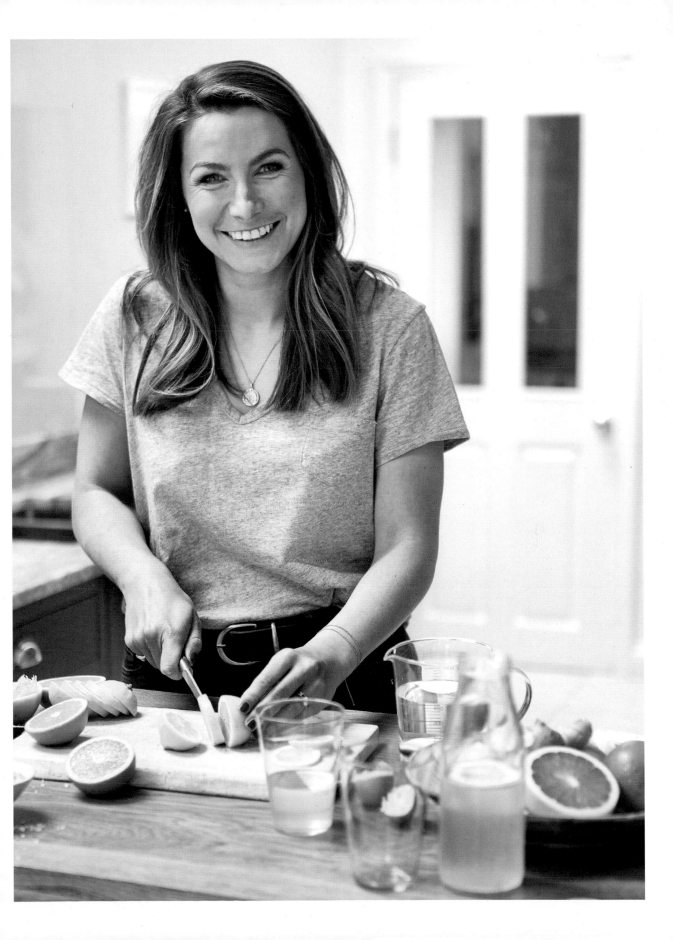

In the beginning, I would get back from a long run and immediately tuck into a packet of chocolate biscuits (usually eating the whole pack) with a cup of tea. Unsurprisingly, I put on weight. I thought that running long distance would mean the pounds just dropped off. But I changed my training completely for my second marathon, completing more speed workouts, cross-training, hitting the gym, and learning more about what to eat. I lost weight during that period, simply from changing my training and eating more mindfully.

In 2013 I ran the New York City Marathon, finishing in 4.09.45 – a 45 minute improvement and on a much hillier course. I've since completed all six Marathon Majors (London, Berlin, Chicago, New York, Tokyo and Boston), earning a Six Star Finisher Medal, and dropped my personal best marathon time to 3.38. I'm hopeful that by the time you read this it will be sub-3.30 or close!

It was around the time of the New York City Marathon that I started to research more about what I should be eating to support my training, and translating what I was learning about nutrition from magazines and websites into healthier meals. I was working at *Good Housekeeping* at the time, writing and testing recipes for the magazine and website, and so my new interest in health found its way into the food, recipes and recommendations we were making in the magazine.

I was also discovering how much mis-information is out there and just how confusing the world of nutrition can be. Few of the blogs I was reading were backed up with any scientific credentials. I discovered that, while anyone can call themselves a 'nutritionist' without any formal credentials, in the UK a dietitian is a protected title. To become a Registered Dietitian you have to complete a three- to four-year degree course. I was fortunate to get some sound advice from Rosie Saunt (co-founder of The Rooted Project and author of *Is Butter a Carb?*), who was training to be a dietitian at the time. I'm forever grateful to her for setting me on the path to becoming a Registered Dietitian myself.

When many people think about dietitians, they often think about helping patients to lose weight or stick to specific diets; they don't always think about those that can't eat. As part of my four-year dietetics degree, I spent six months in a hospital placement. It was during that time at St Mary's Hospital, London, that I discovered the clinical area I wanted to specialize in: intensive care, where a lot of patients need to be tube-fed until they recover enough to eat or can be transferred to long-term care facilities.

I had been nervous about spending time in the intensive care unit (ICU), especially at the trauma centre, because most of their patients were men who had either attempted suicide or had very bad falls. Tragically, I have lost two good friends in this manner and I worried that I wouldn't cope dealing with the patients and families, that it might bring back memories and that I wouldn't be able to do my job. However, a doctor friend asked how I would have wanted Vic and Simon to have been treated if they had made it to intensive care, and so I went into it wanting to do the best job I possibly could. I was there early for daily ward rounds, read extra papers, volunteered to see additional patients and even wrote my dissertation on ICU feeding protocol. I was helped hugely by my ICU mentor Ella Terblanche, one of the most passionate and knowledgeable dietitians I've ever met. I loved the role and I felt I could make a real difference.

When I tell people that I'm studying dietetics, they often ask me about what they should be eating. While every person is different, the one piece of advice I share with everyone is to EAT REAL FOOD. By this, I mean minimally processed foods as close to their natural form as possible.

Ever tried to eat a whole tube of Pringles or a 'sharing bag' of crisps? It's scary how much of a dent you can make in them just by yourself. However, try to over-eat fruit, vegetables or whole grains without any additives and it's much harder. A recent study showed that eating processed foods can actually cause a rise in hunger hormones (such as ghrelin) and increase over-eating. It also showed that participants who ate an unlimited real food diet had higher levels of PYY (a natural appetite-suppressing hormone) and lower levels of ghrelin. They also had a better micronutrient intake.

When I'm training, I often feel as though I eat non-stop and have to ensure that I have easy-to-reach snacks on hand at all times. I'm currently training for a triathlon and swimming hunger is its own beast. Since marathon hunger (or hanger) is real, it makes sense to fuel that hunger (and refuel your muscles and energy systems) with predominantly natural whole foods, a.k.a. 'real food'.

I know that, in reality, our busy, overstretched lives mean that we sometimes reach for convenience foods – the cereal bar from the petrol station, a ready-made salad for lunch or a microwavable meal for dinner after a long day. Sometimes, that really is the best option to fuel our body quickly. However, in this book, I've tried to offer you the real food options.

The 20-Minute Meals chapter (page 68) includes recipes that can be on the table speedily with a limited list of ingredients. The two-week meal plan on pages 26–7 shows you which recipes make great lunch leftovers or make-ahead breakfasts. And the recipes in the Snacks chapter (page 150) have been designed to give you a much-needed energy boost mid-morning or mid-afternoon, while also fuelling your body with protein, carbs and fat for your next workout (or simply to help you recover efficiently from your morning run or gym session). All the recipes have been tested on non-running friends, the kids I nanny and my husband (who is a rather reluctant runner, yet has completed two London Marathons!) and I can assure you that they go down a storm, even without logging a long run first. Although, personally, I think anything tastes better after a couple of miles, especially the Monster Workout Cookies on page 123!

Portion Sizes

I use the 'Eatwell Plate' as a good guideline for portion sizes when it comes to carbohydrates, protein and fat.

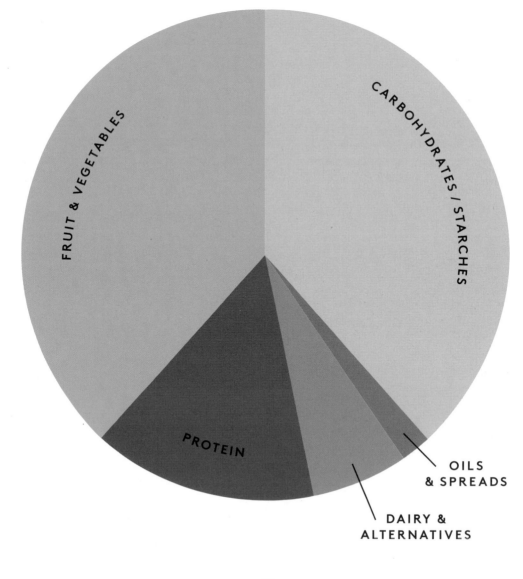

FRUIT & VEGETABLES

CARBOHYDRATES / STARCHES

PROTEIN

OILS & SPREADS

DAIRY & ALTERNATIVES

Personally, I don't count calories. You'll notice that I haven't included calorie counts in this book, with the exception of one chapter: Homemade Running Fuel (page 28). This is because I think it's important that you fuel your runs appropriately and can be sure that you're getting enough calories and carbs for your workout or race.

I have included labels throughout to denote 'High Energy', 'High Fibre' and 'High Protein' recipes, and of course you can feel free to use the ingredients lists to count the calories/macronutrients if you want.

There isn't a 'one rule suits all' approach to nutrition. Each body is different, and needs to be fed differently, although the general rule that you should eat a combination of carbs, fat and protein is universal. Also true for all is the fact that the body thrives best on whole foods with a high nutrient quality. So do what works for you: count calories, track your macros and weigh your food if you find that helpful and not harmful. Just remember that eating should be enjoyable, social and nourishing – try not to lose sight of that.

KEY TO RECIPE SYMBOLS

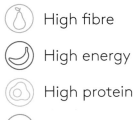

High fibre

High energy

High protein

Vegan

Rest Days

Rest days are a crucial part of training and are actually when most of your 'gains' occur, through the growth of lean muscle. Insulin plays a key role in this, and for insulin to be released into the body we need to eat. When we eat, in particular carbohydrates, glucose is absorbed from our gut into our bloodstream, raising blood glucose levels and signalling to the pancreas to release insulin. If you don't eat enough, then you won't have sufficient insulin for muscle growth and repair.

I like to look at energy balance/calorie intake over a week rather than in individual days. So, while it's important to fuel yourself appropriately for your daily exercise requirements and to fuel your recovery, I tend to eat much the same on rest days as I do on the days that I train.

Additionally, you want to gain the maximum benefits from your rest days, which are for muscle repair, replenishment of glycogen (energy) stores and aiding recovery. In order to do this, you need to consume sufficient carbohydrates and protein.

Ensure you eat good-quality carbohydrates. Whole grains, fruits, vegetables and beans, alongside lean protein from meat, fish, dairy, eggs or plant-based sources, provide the amino acids essential for muscle repair and growth.

Protein

One of three macronutrients, protein is essential for a number of roles within the body. We runners, gym junkies, endurance enthusiasts and fitness fans are probably most concerned with the role that it plays in muscle building and repair. If we refuel and recover properly, the work we do in the gym and on the road and trails will lead to improvements in strength and speed. Yet although the media might have you believe that protein is THE most important macronutrient for those who exercise, I think all three are of equal importance for training and performance, as well as for overall health.

Protein is also important to help stave off 'hanger' – it is arguably the most satiating macronutrient as it takes the longest for the body to digest. It also plays a crucial role in hormone function, in particular insulin, which helps regulate blood sugar levels. Furthermore, insulin is important for the body's breakdown of glucose into energy – pretty crucial to avoid hitting that wall at mile 20!

UK Government guidelines give the average person a requirement of 0.8g of protein per kg of bodyweight per day – around 35 per cent of our diet. But, if you're reading this, you're probably not average. Athletes' requirements are likely to be higher. For runners, that means between 1–1.2g/kg bodyweight/day, and for those who are doing a lot of strength training, that increases to up to 2g/kg bodyweight/day

(according to the American College for Sports Medicine, Dieticians of Canada and the Academy of Nutrition and Dietetics). Ensuring that you have enough protein at each meal (around 20g), and eating it regularly throughout the day with each meal and snack, should keep you full, and will help you meet your daily protein targets.

Without overcomplicating things (because, let's face it, I only learned the names of all the amino acids during my dietetics degree to pass the exam), protein is made up of 21 amino acids, nine of which are known as the essential amino acids. These essential amino acids can't be made in the body and are therefore crucial to obtain from your diet. Complete proteins contain all nine essential amino acids. These are mostly animal proteins (meat, fish, eggs, dairy); however, some plant-based proteins such as quinoa are also 'complete'. Most plant-based proteins are missing a few amino acids, and therefore need to be eaten in combination with other proteins to become complete, e.g. rice and beans, or bread and hummus. This can be done throughout the day, rather than at just one meal; however, I find it easiest to remember them in pairs!

How much protein is there in real food?

Food source	Amount of protein
1 medium egg	6g
1 salmon fillet (100g/3½oz)	25g
1 chicken breast (145g/5oz)	35g
1 steak (200g/7oz)	40g
1 pork loin fillet (100g/3½oz)	22g
small cup of beans/lentils/ chickpeas (garbanzo beans) (125g/4½oz cooked weight)	11g
glass of semi-skimmed milk (200ml/scant 1 cup) (see note)	7.2g
small pot of dairy or soya yoghurt (100g/3½oz/scant ½ cup)	4.1g
broccoli (100g/2 cups chopped)	4.3g
soy beans/edamame (80g/ generous ½ cup)	11.2g
peas (80g/generous ½ cup)	5.4g
nuts (25g/3 Tbsp)	4.8g
seeds (25g/3½ Tbsp)	6.4g

NOTE:

Dairy milk is a great source of protein (and carbs) that is easily digestible in the body (check out the Iced Latte Cubes recipe on page 110 for a delicious recovery drink). However, for various reasons, many people are cutting down on dairy in their diets and swapping milk for dairy-free alternatives. While tasty, they do not deliver the same nutritional content as cows' milk, and most do not contain protein or calcium. Soy milk contains around 6.5g per 200ml (only a little less than dairy), while oat, nut and rice milks contain minimal amounts. Personally, I would recommend choosing unsweetened, fortified dairy-free milks that have added vitamins and minerals rather than 'fresh' nut, oat or rice milks. I keep a stash of long-life oat milk in my cupboard to use in smoothies, baking and porridge, and for times when I've run out of milk for my coffee!

Protein Powders

It can feel as though a protein shake is an essential addition to everyone's gym bag, but if you're eating protein regularly throughout the day, choosing a mixture of protein-rich foods for meals and snacks, then you should be able to meet your protein targets using real food.

However, if you don't feel like you're getting enough protein from your diet, or if you are travelling, training extra hard or just find it tough to get a post-workout snack or recovery meal in, then you could look at adding some protein powder into your diet.

Not all protein powders are created equal, and many have hidden sugars and artificial flavourings added in. There are also a plethora of options, both vegan and non-vegan choices.

WHEY PROTEIN

The most common type of protein is made from whey, a bi-product of the dairy industry. It's a complete protein, meaning it has all nine essential amino acids. Choose between isolate (high levels of protein with very little lactose) and concentrate (cheaper, but higher in lactose, fat and carbohydrates). With speedy absorption rates, whey protein is perfect for quick muscle recovery.

CASEIN PROTEIN

Also a milk derivative, this is broken down slightly more slowly than whey protein, providing a continuous release of amino acid over a longer period of time. If you've come to the end of the day and realize you haven't had enough protein, then casein protein can be a great option to stir into a pudding or yoghurt before bed to provide a steady stream of amino acid overnight.

COLLAGEN PEPTIDES

While there isn't as much research on collagen protein as on other animal proteins, collagen is increasing in popularity, particularly among runners. Collagen is the main protein in our bodies; it's made naturally but production declines as we get older. Collagen peptides act as building blocks for local cells and help boost production of new collagen fibres within the skin, bones and cartilage. This can improve joint health and mobility, as well as strengthen your nails and hair. Probably best when mixed with whey protein, to maximize muscle synthesis and get a fuller range of amino acids.

HEMP PROTEIN

Personally, I think this is the best plant-based protein supplement as it provides all nine of the essential amino-acids. However, the taste alone isn't brilliant, so mix it into a nut butter/chocolate smoothie, or bake it into the Triple Chocolate Banana Bread (page 113) to disguise the flavour.

BROWN RICE PROTEIN

————

Derived from wholegrain rice, this plant-based protein is best in combination with other protein powders (hemp or pea) or milk/eggs to complete the essential amino acid profile. Another option is to mix into smoothies, yoghurt or porridge for a protein boost.

PEA PROTEIN

————

Not a complete protein; however, you can create a complete vegan protein by mixing it with hemp or brown rice protein. Add to smoothies, yoghurt or porridge – the flavour on its own isn't great!

SOY PROTEIN

————

Another plant-based protein with a complete amino acid profile, with only a slightly lower synthesis rate than whey protein. It is high in protein, low in carbohydrates and comes in a variety of flavours, making it a good option to consume mixed with water.

Gluten

————

A question I've heard a lot is whether you need to cut out gluten to improve running performance. Gluten is a protein found in wheat, rye and barley. In most people these proteins are harmless. However, for some, they can cause damage in the small intestine, destroying the lining of your gut. Those diagnosed with coeliac disease have to strictly cut all gluten from their diet. However, for the rest of us, there shouldn't be a need to avoid gluten.

It is true that low numbers of people may be more sensitive to gluten than others (but have not been diagnosed as coeliac), but more research needs to be done in the area. For many, it could be the type of gluten-containing foods that they are eating (e.g. cakes, large bowls of pasta, biscuits, etc.) that are actually the issue, rather than gluten itself. Some scientists also believe that those who have gluten sensitivity may actually just have a different food allergy or intolerance that is yet to be diagnosed.

Carbohydrates

'When athletes compete in endurance events, it is carbohydrates, not fat-based fuels that are the predominant fuel for the working muscles, and carbohydrate, not fat, availability that become rate limiting for performance.'
Hawley and Leckey, *Sports Medicine*, 2015

Recently, carbohydrates seem to have become the most villainized macronutrient, but they are a runner's best friend, providing the largest single source of energy in the diet (between 45–65 per cent of our total diet). Glucose is the muscles' (and brain's) preferred energy source, most of which comes from carbohydrate breakdown. When glycogen (carbohydrate energy) stores are depleted, stored fat can be burned to provide energy.

Typically, when we think of carbs, the first things that come to mind are bread, potatoes, rice, oats and grains; but fruit, vegetables, beans and legumes are also great sources in your diet.

Simple carbohydrates (such as glucose and fructose) are broken down and absorbed quickly into the bloodstream to give a fast energy boost. Real food versions are found in fruit, milk, yoghurt, cakes and juices.

Complex carbohydrates, also known as polysaccharides, are made up of multiple sugar groups linked together. This makes it harder for the body to break them down, slowing down the release of energy into the bloodstream and giving you a longer-lasting energy burn. Examples are potatoes, quinoa or wholegrain rice these are the types of carbs you want to have with most meals to keep your energy levels stable throughout the day, fuelling you through your workout, job, social life and whatever else you tackle. They are also key for longer runs/workouts, typically in combination with simple carbohydrates to replenish glucose when your stores start to get low. An example would be having a bowl of oats and a banana for breakfast before a 14-mile run, then consuming an 'energy gel' at 7 miles to keep you powered up to the end of the run.

While simple and refined carbs (typically 'white' versions, such as white bread and other processed foods) have got a bad reputation, I think there is a place for them in a runner's diet. In particular, simple carbs are beneficial post-workout/race for a quick refuel, and in combination with complex carbohydrates (usually wholegrain) pre-race for a mixture of quick- and slow-release energy.

Glycaemic Index

———————

Often abbreviated to GI, the glycaemic index of a food is a ranking of how quickly it is converted into sugars, and therefore the effect it has on your blood glucose levels. A high GI means a food can be quickly digested, causing a spike in blood glucose (and potentially subsequent dip if not eaten in combination with foods that are rich in lower GI carbohydrate, protein or fat). Low GI foods and drinks have a longer digestion time, gradually increasing blood glucose, helping to keep us full over a prolonged period and hopefully avoiding that 'sugar crash'.

As you might imagine, most of the time low GI foods are best, helping us fuel our days and runs/workouts. However, pre- or post-workout/race, picking a mid- to high-GI food or drink can help can help enhance post-exercise refuelling of muscle glycogen. The recipes in the Refuel – Sweet (page 108) and Refuel – Savoury (page 126) sections include a mixture of mid–high GI foods, including sweet potatoes, rice, honey and starchy vegetables.

Fibre

———————

Soluble fibre is easily digested by our gut bacteria and is found in oats, fruits, legumes and vegetables. As well as forming natural gels that soften stools, it may also help maintain stable blood glucose and healthy cholesterol levels.

Insoluble fibre adds bulk to your stool, making it easier to pass and is found in whole grains, vegetable skins, nuts and seeds. Most fibre-rich foods typically contain both kinds.

UK Government guidelines suggest we should be eating 30g fibre per day, including both soluble and insoluble fibre. However, according to the British Nutrition Foundation, currently most of us aren't meeting these targets, with most women consuming just over 17g per day and men around 20g per day.

The one time I'd be a bit wary of over-indulging on fibre is the night before or the morning of a race. In fact, I know a number of runners who reduce their fibre intake in the 3–5 days prior to their goal marathon. Don't go too crazy when cutting out the roughage from your diet though – you know that the pre-race bathroom visit is crucial for a good race day (overshare!).

Fat

Low fat? Reduced fat? No fat? Full fat?

During the 1980s and 90s, this macronutrient was the 'enemy' of health. Now, thankfully, we're steering away from that mentality and realize how important it is to include fats in our diet. Roughly speaking, fats are broken down into three types: saturated, unsaturated and trans fats (although, in reality, most food sources are a combination of fats in different proportions).

SATURATED FATS

Solid at room temperature. Mostly found in animal products, e.g. meat or cheese, but also coconut oil.

UNSATURATED FATS

Mostly found in oils from plant and fish sources – and generally liquid at room temperature – unsaturated fats are both mono-unsaturated (fat molecules that have 1 unsaturated carbon bond) and poly-unsaturated fats (fat molecules that have more than 1 unsaturated carbon bond), found in combination in olive oil, nut oils, in walnuts and sunflower oil, as well as in oily fish and avocado.

TRANS FATS

Mostly artificially made. Should be consumed in limited amounts.

Fat is essential in the diet, and has a role in vitamin absorption, hormone regulation, and muscle growth and development. It should make up between 20–35 per cent of our calorie intake.

You've probably heard of omega-3 and omega-6 fatty acids: these anti-inflammatory types of fat cannot be made in the body and therefore must be consumed as part of our diet. Omega-3s are found in oily fish (salmon, tuna, mackerel), flaxseeds and walnuts, while omega-6s are found in vegetable oils. Studies have linked omega-3s with reduced risk of heart-disease and stroke, as well as having a role in preventing mental health disorders, such as dementia and depression. Try the Pistachio Crusted Salmon (page 134) or Kara Goucher's Poke Bowl (page 133) for a good portion of omega-3s.

Both carbohydrate and fat are used as fuel during exercise. Carbohydrates are the main fuel for moderate to high intensity exercise with fat providing energy for lower intensity exercise. Some endurance athletes aim to become 'fat adapted', training their bodies to use fat as their main energy source for lower intensity endurance exercise, thereby extending the period they can use their glycogen (carbohydrate) stores and enabling them to work at a higher intensity when needed. We store more fat than carbs in our body (which is why we have to replenish carbohydrates as we run long distance), plus with more calories in fat than carbohydrate, gram for gram, fat can provide energy for hours or even days. Ultra-runners in particular are starting to trial fat adaptation. However, the jury is still out on this one and the research has been done on well-trained athletes. Most professional endurance athletes still use carbohydrates as their main energy source for running. Even with full glycogen stores and topping up with appropriate carbohydrates, both carbohydrate and fat will be used for fuel.

Vitamins and Minerals

Also known as micronutrients, vitamins and minerals cannot be made within our body and therefore must be part of our dietary intake.

We need 13 different vitamins to support growth and other functions within our body. They can be broken down into fat-soluble and water-soluble, and each plays a different role.

Fat-soluble Vitamins: A, D, E, K

These vitamins can be stored in the body for months or years until they need to be utilized, meaning these don't have to be part of your daily diet.

VITAMIN A

Also known as retinol (you might recognise this from beauty products). Vitamin A helps keep the skin and the the lining of your respiratory tract, the gut and the bladder healthy, as well as helping vision in low light. It is essential for the normal functioning of your immune system.

VITAMIN D

You'll find it in oily fish, dairy, eggs and red meat, as well as in fortified breakfast cereals. Vitamin D can also be absorbed transdermally through sunlight. Even those of us who run outside regularly may still be vitamin-D deficient, especially during the winter months, and if using high-factor sunscreen in the summer. The current UK advice is for all adults to take a 10 microgram supplement during autumn (fall) and winter.

VITAMIN E

A fat-soluble vitamin also linked to healthy skin and eyes, as well as normal functioning of the immune system.

VITAMIN K

Essential for blood clotting and wound healing. There may also be a link between vitamin K and bone health and maintenance.

Water-soluble Vitamins: C and B complex

Found in a wide variety of foods, these cannot be stored in the body and it's therefore essential you have an adequate intake from your diet.

VITAMIN C

Found in (bell) peppers, broccoli, sweet potatoes and Brussels sprouts, citrus fruits, kiwi and blackcurrants (as well as other fruits).

B12

B12 is commonly deficient among vegans and runners on plant-based diets as it is not found naturally in many plant foods. However, it is added to fortified breakfast cereals and found in yeast extract (so slather it on, Marmite lovers!). It is naturally found in meat, fish, eggs and dairy, and it is utilized in the body to release energy from food, make red blood cells and keep the nervous system healthy.

Minerals

Minerals are found in non-living matter, such as rocks and earth. They are absorbed into plants, which are eaten by us (or animals) and become part of the food chain. Deficiencies tend to occur when you cut things out of your diet, such as following a vegan or vegetarian diet.

IRON

This seems to be a common deficiency amongst runners, especially female runners. It is found in meat, fish, poultry, eggs, beans, nuts, whole grains, fortified breakfast cereals and green leafy veg. Iron enables red blood cells to carry oxygen around the body and therefore deficiencies can hinder athletic performance. Animal sources of iron are more easily absorbed by the body than plant sources, which leads to increased rates of deficiency among vegans and vegetarians. Try to eat your plant-based iron sources alongside a serving of vitamin C (such as orange juice, broccoli, red (bell) pepper) to aid absorption,

and avoid tannins in tea and coffee an hour before or after, which can reduce absorption.

IODINE

Traditionally, milk in the UK was fortified with iodine; however, the switch away from dairy towards plant-based milks has seen iodine intake decrease and we are beginning to see iodine deficiencies for the first time in many years. An iodine deficiency can lead to thyroid issues, so including it regularly in your diet is important. You'll find it in fish, shellfish, seaweed, dairy products and iodized salt.

CALCIUM

Not only linked to teeth and bones, calcium is also important for muscle contraction. Found in dairy, fortified plant-based milks, leafy green veg, lentils, beans, tofu, chickpeas (garbanzo beans) and canned fish with soft edible bones. Absorption of calcium is linked to vitamin D, so you'll often see supplements combining the two.

A NOTE ON SUPPLEMENTS

This is so very individual that I am not in a position (nor should anyone be) to give blanket advice about supplements. However, there are key micronutrients in which many runners are deficient and you could discuss these with your doctor or dietitian. Alternatively, simply look to add more vitamins into your diet through real food.

Hydration

Taking in fluid during a run, whether it's a race or a training run, is a key issue for a runners. Dehydration, particularly during long runs, is a serious concern. Regular fluid ingestion is crucial to normal body function and sports performance, and so getting your fluid balance right is key.

While exercising, as a result of thermoregulation – the process by which our body tries to cool us down – we lose a lot of body water through sweating. When we don't replace the fluid lost through sweat, then hypohydration occurs – a body water deficit. Even a 2 per cent deficit can impair performance, due to increased heart rate, increased perceived exertion and potential loss of coordination. It can also affect the bowels – a dodgy stomach is something we all want to avoid.

As well as hypohydration, athletes are also at risk of hyponatraemia, which causes a sodium dilution in the blood. This occurs when athletes over-hydrate during exercise, and is particularly common in those that are out running for a longer time.

Hydration tips

- Start hydrated. We should be drinking 6–8 glasses of water per day, although if you're living in a hot climate or exercising intensely, this will be greater. Typically around 35ml per kg of bodyweight is what we use to calculate how much fluid you need to drink per day.

- You can use urine colour as an indicator of hydration status: clear straw or light yellow is the aim.

- In general, runs under 1 hour shouldn't require fluid intake (if you're sufficiently hydrated already and it's not very hot).

- For longer runs or particularly intense workouts, either water or an electrolyte drink can help you stay hydrated.

- A 'little and often' approach is usually best during a race.

- If it's hotter than you're used to on a training run or race day, dress appropriately and slow your pace, as even increasing your fluid intake won't necessarily cool you down.

- Don't 'bulk drink' before you run – the body simply cannot absorb it. Between 300–600ml (10–20fl oz/1¼–2½ cups), taken an hour or two before your race/run, should be sufficient, especially when combined with mid-race fluid intake.

- Try to drink around 500ml (17fl oz/generous 2 cups) fluid within 30 minutes of finishing your workout.

- **Don't ignore thirst during a race. If in doubt, drink to thirst.**

Hydration, like nutrition, is individualized. Kenyan runners, for instance, are very well adapted to run with little fluid intake but remain hydrated. As well as your genetics, environment, weather, intensity of exercise and metabolic rate all have an impact on your hydration needs. If you work out your sweat rate you can roughly establish the amount of fluid you need to take in during a run.

HOW TO CALCULATE YOUR SWEAT RATE

1. Record your pre-run weight in kg.

2. Run for 60 minutes without drinking anything.

3. Record your post-run weight in kg.

4. Subtract your post-run figure from your pre-run figure and multiply the result by 1000. The resulting number is the amount of fluid in grams that you lost during your run.

Remember that weather, exertion/pace, time of day etc., will affect the result, so it's worth removing your clothes when weighing and trying to replicate your race conditions if you're working out a race-hydration strategy.

Water or Sports (Electrolyte) Drinks?

When you sweat, you lose crucial electrolytes, particularly sodium, chloride potassium and magnesium. Not only do these electrolytes play a role in maintaining body fluid balance, they are also involved in muscle contraction (which could be one of many reasons why you can experience cramps during a race) and neurological activity.

While we replace electrolytes naturally through the food and fluids we ingest, research has found that drinks containing sodium and carbohydrates increase water absorption in the bloodstream, which is particularly important when you're sweating heavily. You can drink electrolyte drinks during exercise of over 60 minutes or post-workout. Many energy gels also contain electrolytes along with high carbohydrate concentrations, and therefore taking these with water is sufficient (and often more palatable).

What type of drinks to look for:

HYPOTONIC

These drinks are more dilute than your body fluids, meaning they will be absorbed faster than water. The homemade sports drinks on page 45 are designed to be hypotonic to aid absorption and hydration.

ISOTONIC

These are the same concentration as bodily fluids and are therefore absorbed at around the same speed as water. Typically, they contain higher carbohydrate levels than hypotonic drinks, generally around 1.5–2 times more. Most store-bought sports drinks are isotonic, and help the body refuel and rehydrate simultaneously.

HYPERTONIC

Fruit juices and fizzy drinks are more concentrated than bodily fluids, and therefore have a slower rate of absorption and fluid replacement than water. It's better to take these post-run as an energy source, rather than use them for hydration.

Caffeine

Caffeine is a controversial topic, and you're either someone who can drink a cup of coffee pre-race, or you're not.

Caffeine works as a stimulant within the body and can have physiological effects that improve athletic performance beyond the 'wake up' effect on your brain. Studies have shown that it can help reduce perceived effort in exertion at high intensity (so it's perfect for those early morning speed workouts).

Caffeine can enhance mental alertness, reaction time and improve neuromuscular connection, making your muscles fire more efficiently.

For endurance exercise, 3–6mg of caffeine per kg of body weight is recommended, with more profound benefits experienced when you abstain from caffeine several days before you work out (for instance, before a goal race). Elite runner Ryan Hall used to only drink coffee on his key workout and race days to feel the full benefits. However, if you're used to drinking a morning cup daily, then you may feel some adverse effects cutting down. Consuming

your caffeine 45 minutes pre-run/workout has the best impact on performance, however the stimulatory effects can last for up to 6 hours.

Many runners use caffeine mid-race, and it's found in many gels, gums and sports beans. My advice on this would be to practise before using it on a race day, and start sparingly so that you don't experience any negative consequences on the day.

Also, remember that sleep is our best recovery tool, so do try to avoid caffeine too late in the day.

Store-Cupboard Staples

In this book, I've tried to keep it really simple and utilize ingredients that are easily found at your local supermarket/market and which don't require a trip to multiple health food stores to track down (with perhaps the exception of the baobab powder on page 138). For me, the key to choosing healthy meals and snacks is having a good supply of quality foods at home, in the refrigerator, freezer and store cupboard.

Store-cupboard staples

- Oats (I prefer old-fashioned jumbo oats)
- Canned pulses and beans (for quick carbohydrate and protein sources)
- Canned tomatoes
- Coconut milk
- Nut butter (whichever type you like most, but try to choose one without added salt and sugar)
- Wholegrain pasta
- Canned fish
- Spices (my most used are paprika and cinnamon, but having a selection adds flavour to even the most basic meals)
- Garlic
- Lemons/limes

- Soy sauce
- Stock (bouillon) cubes (ideally low sodium)
- Grains (e.g. quinoa, freekeh, bulgur wheat)
- Wholegrain rice
- Fortified dairy-free milk (long-life)
- Olive oil or avocado oil
- Balsamic vinegar

Refrigerator staples

- Milk or dairy-free milk alternative (see also Note on page 13)
- Onions
- Selection of seasonal vegetables
- Selection of seasonal fruit
- Sweet potatoes/white potatoes
- Salad (lettuce, tomatoes, cucumber)
- Crudités (carrots, celery, cucumber) for snacking
- Dips (such as hummus, guacamole or salsa, for dipping and adding to salads/packed lunches)
- Lean protein (e.g. eggs, cooked chicken/turkey, tofu, Quorn)
- Yoghurt (I use Greek yoghurt for added protein, but use plant-based if you prefer)
- Chillies
- Fresh herbs

Meal Plans

When marathon training, I find it's helpful to create weekly meal plans. This ensures that you don't realise at 10p.m. on a Saturday night that you don't have your pre-run breakfast for the morning. It also eliminates the 'what are we going to have for dinner' dilemma that I think everyone has with themselves or their partners/ housemates. Marathon training also takes up a lot of time, so I've created a whole chapter on speedy 20-Minute Meals (page 68), and suggest utilizing leftovers wherever you can to reduce your time and effort in the kitchen.

This 2-week plan is just a suggestion and can be edited to include your favourite weekly pizza night, shop-bought lunches or meals out. It is based around a long run on a Sunday, with a carb-loading dinner on Saturday night and a fuelling breakfast, but feel free to swap this around to suit your training schedule (and life!).

Freezer essentials

- Frozen peas/sweetcorn
- Frozen berries
- Frozen prawns (shrimp) (a quick, lean protein source)
- Fresh pasta (for the speediest meal when you just can't wait 15 minutes)
- Herbs (don't waste fresh herbs when they start to wilt, chop and freeze them ready to add to a pasta sauce, stew or pie filling)
- Wholewheat bread (toasted from frozen is always an option)
- Milk (because if there's ever a time when I can't make a cup of tea at home, I will go into full meltdown)

WEEK 1

	MONDAY	**TUESDAY**	**WEDNESDAY**
BREAKFAST	Teff Pancakes (page 52)	Overnight Oats (page 56)	leftover Teff Pancakes (page 52)
LUNCH	Poke Bowl (page 133)	leftover Hummus Budhha Bowl (page 137)	Deena's Sandwich (page 137)
DINNER	Hummus Buddha Bowl (page 137)	Turkey Burgers (page 72)	Prawn and Pineapple Fajitas (page 86)

WEEK 2

	MONDAY	**TUESDAY**	**WEDNESDAY**
BREAKFAST	Chocolate PB Granola with Yoghurt and Fruit (page 67)	Overnight Oats (page 56)	Oat Berry Bar (page 59)
LUNCH	leftover Roast Chicken (page 142) and veggies	Winter Salad (page 96)	leftover Chorizo Chilli (page 130)
DINNER	Tomato Poached Eggs (page 78)	Chorizo Chilli (page 130)	Fast Fish Tacos (page 83)

THURSDAY	FRIDAY	SATURDAY	SUNDAY
Savoury Quinoa Porridge (page 64)	Breakfast Pizza (page 51)	Mediterranean Eggs (page 60)	Porridge with Chia Jam (page 66)
Mexican Bean Salad (page 84)	leftover Mexican Bean Salad (page 84)	leftover Cheat's Paella (page 76)	leftover Beetroot Curry (page 95)
Cheat's Paella (page 76)	Balinese Beetroot Curry (page 95)	Avocado Carbonara (page 90)	Roast Chicken with Wedges (page 142)

THURSDAY	FRIDAY	SATURDAY	SUNDAY
Egg Muffins (page 169)	Two-Ingredient Pancakes (page 55)	Broccoli and Sweetcorn Fritters (page 63)	Breakfast Baked Sweet Potato (page 48)
Coronation Chickpea Salad (page 103)	Coronation Chickpea Wrap (page 103)	leftover Pistachio-Crusted Salmon (page 134) with salad and potatoes	Thai Veggie Curry Soup (page 140)
Beef and Broccoli Stir-Fry (page 79)	Pistachio-Crusted Salmon (page 134)	Kathrine Switzer's Prawn Pasta (page 100)	Burger Bowl (page 146)

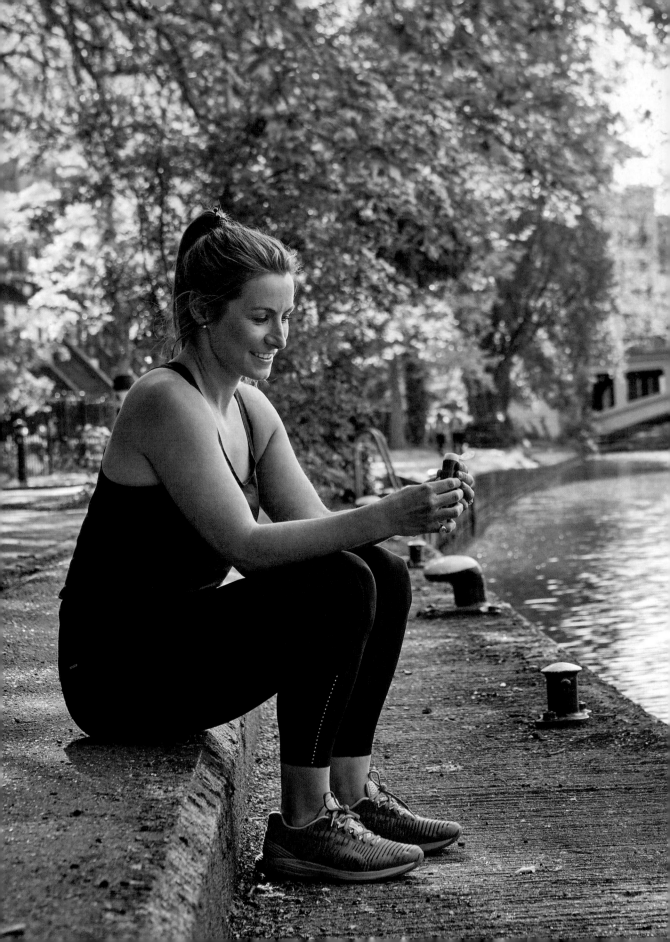

HOMEMADE RUNNING FUEL

As endurance athletes, we must get our fuelling needs, both before and after runs, sorted. But perhaps the hardest fuelling to get right is mid-training/mid-race nutrition. Studies show that there are improvements in performance when taking on carbs during exercise over 60 minutes in duration, as this is the point when depleting glycogen stores start to affect performance. However, if we wait for 60 minutes before refuelling, those glycogen stores will already be getting low, so we need to start fuelling earlier on in the training/race. Even if you don't yet feel low in energy, it's important to start taking on fuel – it will benefit you later in the race, when you might find it harder to stomach.

I know a lot of runners don't get on that well with gels, and yet there aren't many other convenient options available, short of packing yourself a mid-race picnic. Sports nutrition products are designed for fast absorption and ease while out on your run, but part of the reason these gels and specially formulated drinks work so well is the combination of carbohydrate sources they combine. The body can't absorb more than 60g (2oz) of carbohydrates per hour, if ingesting it from a single source. However, if you mix your carbohydrate sources, you can absorb up to 90g (3oz).

For this reason, many of the recipes I have included in this chapter combine sugar and other carbohydrate sources – not to try to make them sickly sweet, but to make them more easily utilized by the body. I also use a lot of coconut water, which is basically nature's sports-performance nectar, containing a mixture of glucose, sucrose and fructose, plus the electrolytes potassium and sodium.

The reality is, if you're eating 'real' food or homemade energy gels when running, you will need to ingest more per hour for maximum benefit. However, I hope that these recipes are a little more palatable for you to enjoy – not to mention cheaper – than most of the gels on the market. It's all about what works for you and your body – whether that's gels, chews, 'real' food, bars or drinks.

GENERAL FUELLING RULES

Run duration	Needs
Under 1 hour	no fuel needed; water if it's hot
1–3 hours	30–60g (1–2oz)
3 hours +	30–90g (1–3oz) carbs per hour (depending on what works for your body!)

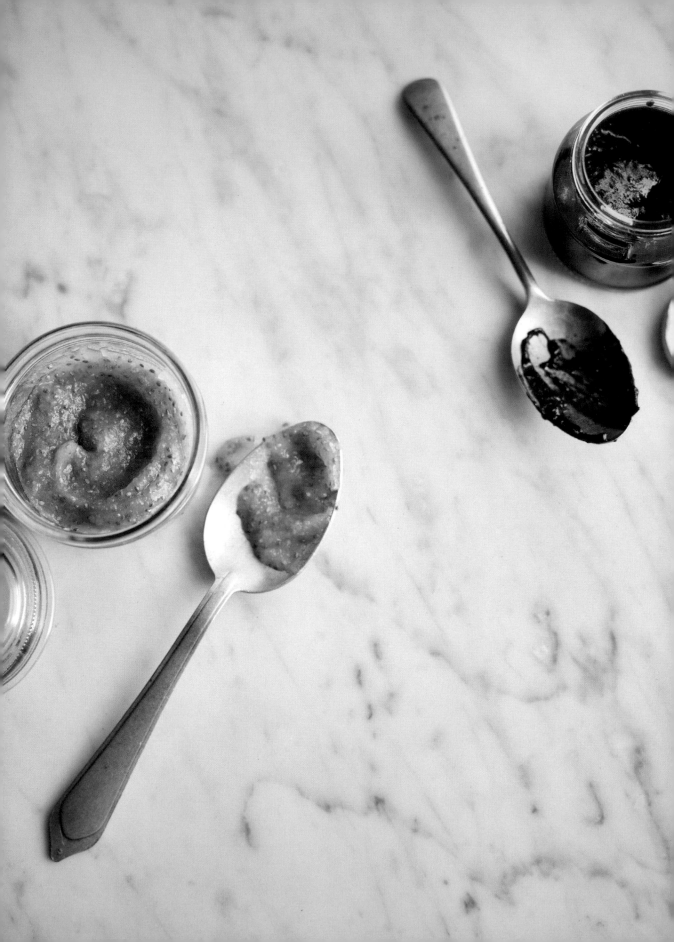

Apple Chia Gels

One of my favourite store-bought energy gels is the Huma apple and cinnamon-flavoured chia gel. Sadly, it doesn't seem to be available everywhere, so I set about making my own. This gel is less convenient to carry, but is definitely cheaper and only takes 15 minutes to make. I use Braeburn apples for their sweet and tart flavour; if you are using cooking apples, add extra maple syrup.

MAKES 400G/14OZ (14 SERVINGS)

2 apples, peeled and
   roughly chopped
75ml (2½fl oz/5 Tbsp)
   unsweetened apple juice
1 Tbsp fresh lemon juice
1 Tbsp maple syrup
2 Tbsp chia seeds
pinch of ground cinnamon
pinch of salt

Put the apples into a large saucepan, cover with a lid and cook over a medium heat, stirring regularly, until they start to break down and become soft.

Remove from the heat, add the apple juice, lemon juice, maple syrup and chia seeds and use a hand-held blender to blitz until smooth. Alternatively, blend in a food processor. Season to taste with cinnamon and salt.

Chill until ready to use; the gel will keep for up to a week in the refrigerator or in the freezer for up to 3 months. The mixture can be placed in small lidded containers to be eaten with a spoon, or decanted into squeezy gel tubes to be eaten on the go. It also works really well as a toast topping!

Fruit Smoothie Gels

Basically a thick fruit smoothie, this homemade gel can be stored in reusable squeezy tubes (these can be found in camping shops, online or I've also found some at Muji – a good place to start is looking at refillable cosmetics tubes). They are a little harder to fit into the pockets of your leggings than traditional gels, but are zero-waste and taste better! You'll need two of these homemade gels for every one traditional gel (each contains about 60 calories and 15g ($\frac{1}{2}$oz) of carbohydrates).

MAKES 500G/1LB 2OZ (14 SERVINGS)

350g (12oz/2¾ cups) frozen blueberries
100g (3½oz/scant 1 cup) frozen raspberries
170g (6oz/1 cup) Medjool dates, pitted and roughly chopped
4–5 Tbsp maple syrup
pinch of salt

Combine the frozen fruit and dates in a large saucepan over a medium heat. Cook for 20–25 minutes, stirring every few minutes to stop the fruit sticking to the bottom of the pan. Allow to cool slightly.

Transfer the cooked fruit to a blender along with the maple syrup and salt and blitz until smooth. Let cool completely, then divide the mixture among freezer bags or squeezy gel tubes to be eaten on the go. Freeze what you're not using immediately and keep for up to 1 month and refrigerate the rest for up to 1 week.

EAT LIKE AN ELITE

Molly Huddle's Tart Cherry Jelly

American distance runner Molly Huddle placed fourth in the New York City Marathon 2018 with a time of 2:26:44. She competed in the 2016 Rio Olympics, setting the American record for 10,000 metres and finishing in sixth place. Molly loves tart cherry jelly (jello). Studies have shown that tart cherries are a great source of antioxidants and can help promote sleep when taken before bed due to their naturally occurring melatonin. For some runners, taking tart cherry juice – such as Montmorency Cherry Juice/ Cherry Active concentrate – before a marathon, reduces damage, soreness and inflammation both during and after the race.

MAKES 18 SQUARES

2 tsp agar powder
   (3 Tbsp agar-agar flakes)
400ml (13fl oz/1⅔ cups)
   pure cherry juice
6 Tbsp Cherry Active
   concentrate
2 Tbsp maple syrup
pinch of salt

Heat the agar and cherry juice in a small saucepan over a medium-high heat. Bring to the boil, then reduce to a simmer and cook for 5 minutes.

Remove from the heat and stir in the cherry active concentrate, maple syrup and salt until dissolved.

Line a 900g (2lb) loaf tin (pan) with cling film (plastic wrap). Pour the mixture into the tin and leave at room temperature for 2–4 hours, or until set.

Turn out and cut into 18 squares.

Store in the refrigerator for up to 2 weeks.

NOTE

The jelly recipes in this chapter are set with agar, to ensure they keep their structure. The texture isn't as pleasing to eat, but you don't end up with a soggy mess halfway through a long run.

Salted Watermelon Squares

Inspired by my favourite Margarita Shot Bloks, these could not be simpler. Unfortunately, the benefits of tequila for runners have not yet been proved, so I use watermelon juice instead. Watermelon contains L-Citrulline, an amino acid involved with nitric oxide synthesis (a gas that widens blood vessels) and glucose transportation into the skeletal muscle, which studies have linked to improvements in athletic performance.

With 36 calories and 8.7g ($\frac{1}{3}$oz) of carbohydrates in these salty squares, you might want to take two to three in place of a regular gel, typically every 30–60 minutes.

MAKES 12

1 tsp agar powder (1½ Tbsp agar-agar flakes)
300ml (10fl oz/1¼ cups) watermelon juice
4 Tbsp caster (superfine) sugar
large pinch of salt

In a large saucepan, mix together the agar powder and watermelon juice over a medium-high heat. Bring to the boil, then reduce to a simmer and cook for 5 minutes.

Line a 450g (1lb) loaf tin (pan) with cling film (plastic wrap).

Remove from the heat and stir in the sugar and salt. Pour the mixture into the tin and leave to set at room temperature for 30–45 minutes or in the refrigerator for 15 minutes.

Turn out and cut into 12 large squares.

Store in the refrigerator for up to 2 weeks.

Cheat's Jelly Shots

These are quick, cheap and easy to make. I also find them really refreshing to eat on a run. With about 40 calories in each square, you'll want to eat three of these shots in place of a gel, or nibble on them more frequently than you would usually fuel. I typically eat three of these every 4–5 miles (6.5–8km) during a full marathon or long run, or every 3–4 miles (5–6.5km) during a half marathon or middle-distance run.

MAKES 20

600ml (20fl oz/2½ cups)
    coconut water
2 tsp agar powder
    (3 Tbsp agar-agar flakes)
50g (2oz/¼ cup) caster
    (superfine) sugar
1 x 135-g (4¾oz) packet
    flavoured jelly (jello)
    cubes (not sugar-free)
large pinch of salt

Place 300ml (10fl oz/1¼ cups) of the coconut water and the agar into a large saucepan and simmer for 5 minutes. Remove from the heat, then stir in the sugar and jelly (jello) cubes. Continue stirring until the jelly cubes have completely melted, then stir in the remaining coconut water and salt.

Line a 20-cm (8-in) square cake tin (pan) with cling film (plastic wrap). Pour the mixture into the tin and chill in the refrigerator overnight.

Turn out and cut into 2.5–4-cm (1–1½-in) squares.

Store in the refrigerator for up to 2 weeks.

NOTE FOR U.S. READERS

A standard 3-oz packet of jello cubes will set 2 cups of liquid, so either reduce the quantity of coconut water to suit or use $1\frac{1}{4}$ packets of jello.

Electrolyte Energy Squares

Use your favourite electrolyte hydration mix to make these jelly (jello) squares. I use Nuun Performance, which contains a mix of electrolytes and carbohydrates.

With about 30 calories and 7g ($\frac{1}{4}$oz) of carbohydrates in each square, you'll want to eat three to four of these in place of a gel, or nibble on them more frequently than you would usually fuel. Their jelly-like texture makes them easier to eat and swallow than a typical chewy block, and I think they are easier to manage than a gel (especially when taken without water).

MAKES 12

1 tsp agar powder (1½ Tbsp agar-agar flakes)
2 electrolyte tablets or 2 servings of electrolyte powder
4 Tbsp caster (superfine) sugar

In a large saucepan, mix together 200ml (7fl oz/scant 1 cup) of water with the agar over a medium-high heat. Bring to the boil, then reduce to a simmer and cook for 5 minutes.

In a small bowl, dissolve the electrolyte tablets/powder in 100ml (3½fl oz/scant ½ cup) cold water.

Line a 450-g (1-lb) loaf tin (pan) with cling film (plastic wrap).

Remove the agar mixture from the heat and stir in the sugar and the electrolyte mixture. Pour into the tin and leave to set at room temperature for 30–45 minutes or in the refrigerator for 15 minutes.

Turn out and cut into 12 large squares.

Store in the refrigerator for up to 2 weeks.

Super Stuffed Dates

No time to leave anything to set or cool? Whip these up in two minutes with ingredients from your storecupboard. You can make as many or as few as you want of these. They also make a great mid-afternoon sweet treat or snack, as do the Berry Chia Bites, pictured opposite (page 40).

These are the most energy-dense of the homemade fuels, with 75 calories and 11g ($\frac{1}{3}$oz) of carbohydrates in each serving (or more, depending on how generous you are with your nut butter filling!).

MAKES AS MANY
AS YOU LIKE

dried pitted dates
sunflower seed butter or
  a favourite nut butter
sea salt, to taste

Prise open each date and
spoon in ½ teaspoon of your
chosen butter (be careful
not to overstuff). Sprinkle
with a little salt and close
the date around the
stuffing. If you want
to make them more
solid for your run, you
can freeze them.

Berry Chia Bites

Personally, I think these are the best-tasting of all the 'on-the-run' fuels – they taste like solid jam! My friend Emily (who I ran my first ever marathon alongside, when we didn't fuel at all!) is a jam monster, and I know she would approve.

With just over 40 calories per bite, you're going to want to either snack on these every 15 minutes or so, or eat three to four every 30–60 minutes, but as always practise during training runs to see what works best for you.

MAKES 20–25 SQUARES

250g (9oz/2 cups) frozen or fresh raspberries
juice of 1 lemon
100g (3½oz/½ cup) caster (superfine) sugar
75g (2⅔oz/5 Tbsp) chia seeds
2 Tbsp agar-agar flakes
½ tsp baking powder

Heat the raspberries in a medium saucepan over a low heat, mashing them until completely softened and of a spoonable consistency. Stir in the lemon juice, sugar and 100ml (3½fl oz/ 7 Tbsp) water, increase the heat and bring to the boil. Add the chia seeds, agar-agar flakes and baking powder and cook, stirring, for 1 minute (the mixture will bubble a lot), then reduce the heat to a simmer. Cook for a further 5–8 minutes, stirring regularly to avoid the chia seeds sticking to the bottom of the pan.

Line a 23-cm (9-in) square cake tin (pan) with cling film (plastic wrap). Pour the mixture into the tin and chill in the refrigerator for 3 hours.

Turn out and cut into 2.5-cm (1-in) squares.

Store in the refrigerator for up to 3 weeks.

Salted Caramel Balls

For years, I've used salted caramel gels for my long runs and races. As someone who sweats a lot, I appreciate the extra salt content, plus they're one of the only flavours I can handle after running for more than 3 hours. These salted caramel balls are more natural than gels, taste a lot better and are perfect for popping into your backpack or pocket to enjoy mid-run for a little energy boost – just make sure they are well wrapped.

MAKES 16 BALLS

50g (2oz/½ cup) rolled
   (old-fashioned) oats
8 Medjool dates, pitted
120g (4¼oz/1 cup) cashews
50g (2oz/generous ⅓ cup)
   whole almonds
2 tsp vanilla extract
large pinch of sea salt

Blitz the oats in a food processor until they are a fine consistency. Add the dates, cashews, almonds, vanilla and salt, then pulse until the mixture comes together and is thick and sticky in texture (add a little water if it is too dry).

Roll the mixture into 16 balls and transfer to a lined baking sheet. Freeze the balls for at least 3 hours.

When ready to use, the frozen balls can be transferred to an airtight container, ziplock bag or your running backpack. They can be stored in the freezer for up to 3 months.

Drinks

One of the best pieces of hydration advice I received from a coach is that if you're thirsty during your first rep of a speed workout, or the first mile, then you aren't drinking enough throughout the day. You shouldn't need to drink during your speed session, unless it's particularly hot.

In general, runs under 1 hour shouldn't require fluid intake mid-run; however, if you do want to drink, water is sufficient.

For longer runs, a sports drink containing a mix of electrolytes and carbohydrates helps rehydrate and fuel the body. During very hot sessions or runs lasting longer than 2 hours, make sure there's enough sodium in the drink to account for sweating (ever felt that crusty salty face? Yep, that's you losing sodium).

The problem with many shop-bought electrolyte or 'energy' drinks, is that they are packed with sugar and more calories than you actually need during/post workout. These drinks contain 55–70 calories and 12–17g ($\frac{1}{2}$–$\frac{2}{3}$oz) of carbohydrates per serving.

Have a look at pages 108–49 for what to eat/drink for the best post-workout recovery.

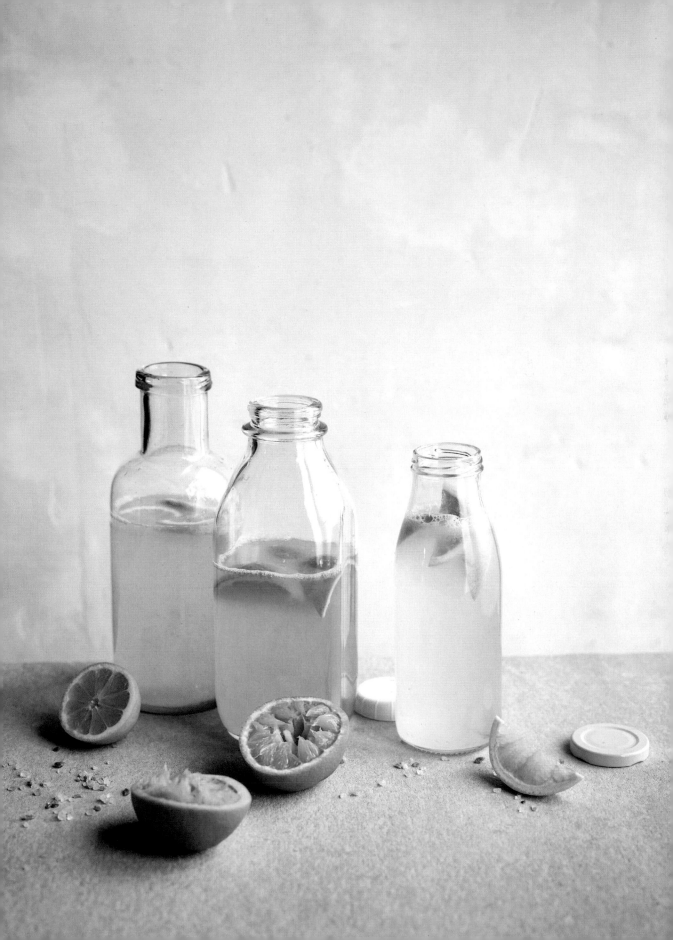

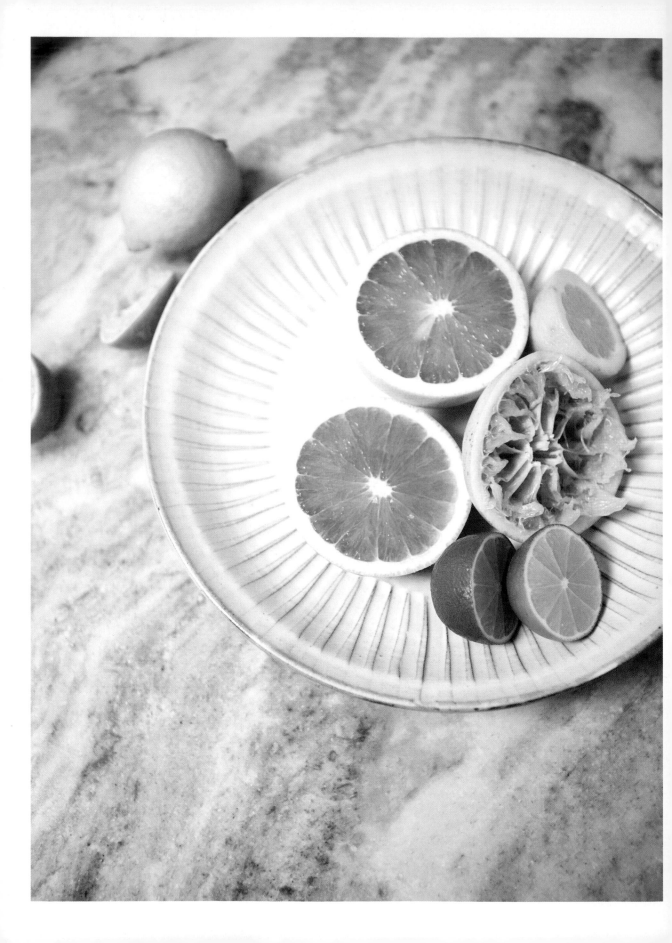

Grapefruit Electrolyte Drink

SERVES 2 (MAKES 500ML/ 17FL OZ/GENEROUS 2 CUPS)

1 Tbsp raw honey or manuka honey
100ml (3½fl oz/7 Tbsp) fresh grapefruit juice
    (about ½ grapefruit, squeezed)
pinch of sea salt or Himalayan salt

Bring 3½ Tbsp of water to the boil and stir in the honey until dissolved. Stir in the grapefruit juice, then add another 350ml (12fl oz/1½ cups) cold water. Stir in a pinch of salt and chill until ready to drink. It will keep for up to 3 days in the refrigerator.

Orange Drink

SERVES 2 (MAKES 500ML/ 17FL OZ/GENEROUS 2 CUPS)

juice of 1 large orange
    (about 100ml/3½fl oz/7 Tbsp)
1 tsp maple syrup (or honey)
250ml (8½fl oz/generous 1 cup) coconut water
pinch of salt (optional)

Squeeze the orange juice into a large jug, then, if using, stir in the maple syrup until dissolved. Mix in the coconut water and a pinch of salt (if using), then dilute with 150–200ml (5–7fl oz/⅔–scant 1 cup) cold water, to taste. Chill until ready to drink. It will keep for up to 2 days in the refrigerator.

Lemon Ginger Drink

SERVES 2–3 (MAKES 560ML/ 19FL OZ/2⅓ CUPS)

thumb-sized piece of fresh root ginger,
    finely grated
juice of 1 lemon
2 Tbsp fresh orange juice
2 Tbsp agave nectar
pinch of sea salt or Himalayan salt

Combine the ginger and the lemon and orange juices in a large jug. Add the agave nectar, salt and 500ml (17fl oz/generous 2 cups) water and stir until the agave nectar and salt have completely dissolved. Sieve (strain) the mixture into a large bottle or glass and chill until ready to drink. It will keep for up to 3 days in the refrigerator.

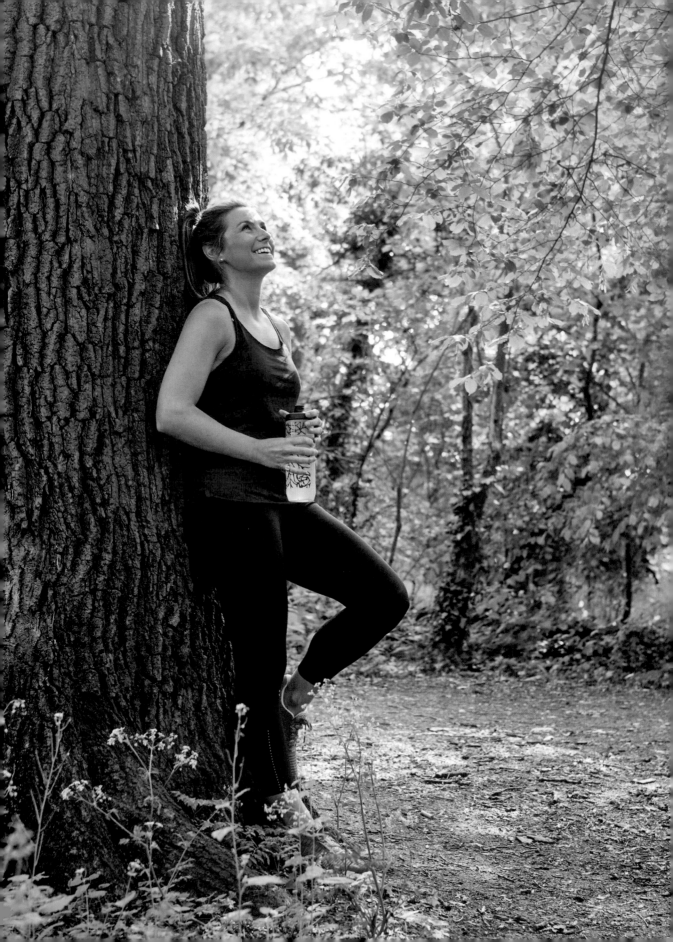

BREAKFAST

'Breakfast is the most important meal of the day.'

Did you know that the cereal manufacturer Kellogg's was more than likely to have funded the study that made this phrase famous? In fact, during the course of my dietetics degree, the NHS has changed its recommendations: it has gone from promoting breakfast as a weight-stabilizing/loss tip for all, to letting those that report to never having breakfast continue that way. It has been found that encouraging people to have breakfast means you simply add calories to their diets rather than taking them away from another meal or snack.

However, if – like me – you are an early-morning runner, both for shorter weekday sessions and weekend long runs, then breakfast truly could be the most important meal of the day.

For the majority of my runs, including speed and tempo workouts, I run on an empty stomach or just have a milky coffee. This means that breakfast is the post-run refuel that my body needs. I combine carbohydrates, protein and fat into my morning meal (see page 10 for the perfect refuel ratio). Typically, I grab a pot of pre-prepared Overnight Oats (page 56) or an Oat Berry Breakfast Bar (page 59) for after my 'Track Tuesday' workouts. The Porridge (page 64) and Two-Ingredient Pancakes (page 55) come together surprisingly quickly for a mid-week morning brekkie, whilst the Teff Pancakes (page 52) can be cooked in batches and frozen and toasted for a speedy start.

On Saturdays, I love to do parkrun (a free, timed 5K in my local park – now an international organisation; find your nearest parkrun at www.parkrun.org.uk) followed by a big breakfast. In the past, that would have been a hungover fry-up... now it's more likely to be Broccoli and Sweetcorn Fritters with poached eggs (page 63) or Mediterranean Eggs (page 60). Oh, how times have changed!

Sundays are for long runs and races. On these mornings, I typically opt for something with a higher carbohydrate content, such as porridge, Breakfast Baked Sweet Potatoes (page 48) or a Breakfast Pizza (page 51). My top tip is to try to have the same thing to eat before your long runs as you're going to have on race day. You want to avoid too much fibre or fat to avoid the dreaded porta-loo dash.

Ideally, you want to take on 400–500 calories, about 2–3 hours before a race (I typically leave less time than this during training runs). Studies have shown that combining protein with carbohydrates before endurance sport can promote muscle repair while exercising, so all of my breakfasts include a protein source, such as milk, nut butter, oats or eggs.

Breakfast Baked Sweet Potatoes

If you're in a hurry, you can microwave the sweet potato for 5–10 minutes, turning it regularly or bake it the night before and reheat before your run. Alternatively, cut the sweet potato into slices 5mm ($\frac{1}{4}$in) thick, and grill (broil) on high for 5 minutes, or until cooked through. Spread the nut butter over the slices and top with banana and cacao nibs.

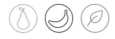

SERVES 1

1 medium sweet potato,
   thoroughly cleaned
1 Tbsp crunchy peanut butter
1 medium banana
1 tsp cacao nibs or chia seeds
   (optional)

TOP TIP

I usually bake a few sweet potatoes at once to have as a quick lunch, breakfast or baking fuel ready to go.

Preheat the oven to 200°C/400°F/gas mark 6.

Using a fork or skewer, poke a number of holes into the sweet potato. Lay it on a baking sheet and roast for 45 minutes–1 hour, or until the insides are soft and a skewer can be easily inserted.

Carefully remove the potato from the oven and slice in half. Split the potato open and dollop the peanut butter into the middle, then close it up slightly while you cut the banana to let the butter melt.

Cut the banana into slices and lay them on top of the potato halves, then top with a sprinkling of cacao nibs or chia seeds, if using. Serve immediately.

SUPERFOOD: BANANAS

Not only are bananas a great source of carbohydrates (there's 27g/1oz of carbs in the average banana), they are a low-glycemic-index carb that releases energy slowly, making it the perfect pre-race/long-run fuel. They are easy to travel with, can be purchased anywhere and can be nibbled on as you wait for your race to start. However, one of the key reasons they are perfect for runners is their electrolyte content. They are a great source of potassium and magnesium, key electrolytes we lose when we sweat. Consuming potassium can help prevent cramps, and it is also involved with fluid balance and nerve impulses (including heart rate), whilst magnesium is involved with muscle function, immune support, energy metabolism and protein synthesis.

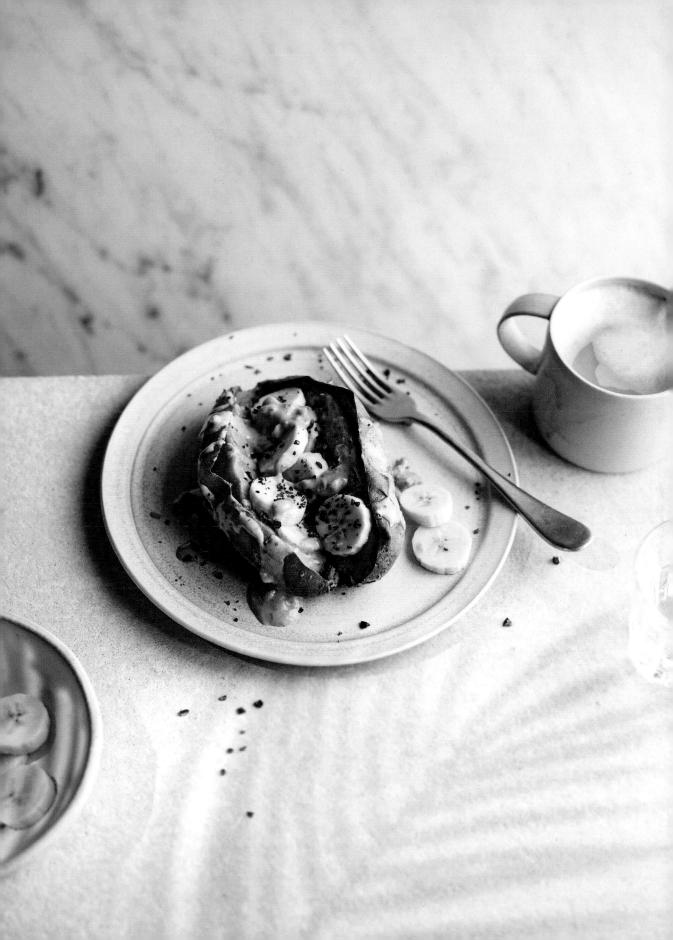

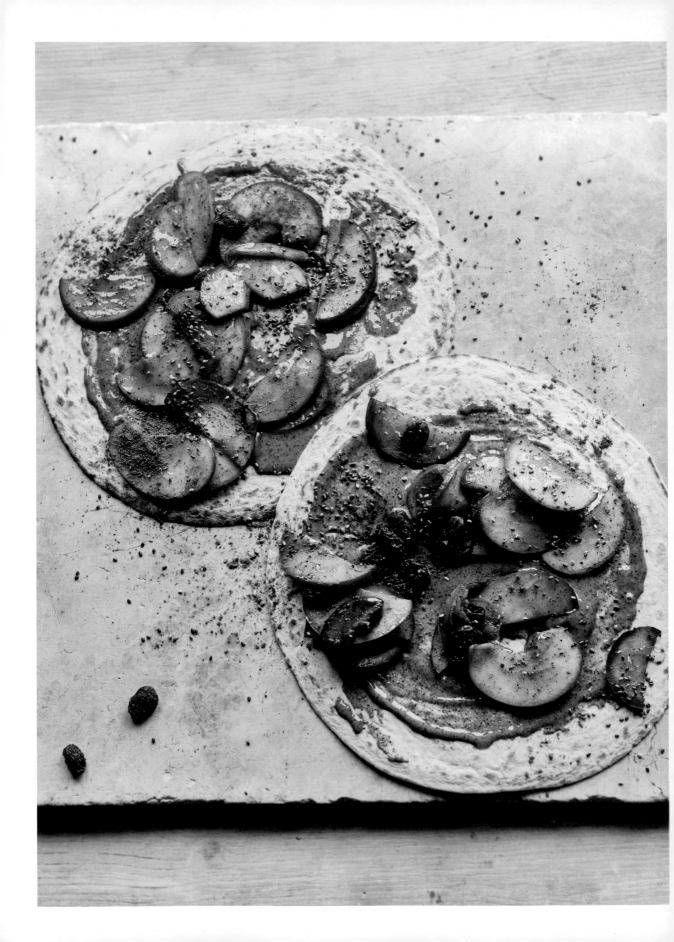

Breakfast Pizza

Bored of peanut butter and bananas on toast? This wrap, topped with almond butter and warm apple slices, not only smells and tastes amazing, but is the ideal pre-long-run fuel for chilly autumn/winter miles. It also makes a great afternoon snack before a big workout. Simply microwave the apple, sultanas (golden raisins), lemon juice, honey and cinnamon in 20-second blasts, until the apples are softened and warmed through. Warm the tortilla and assemble!

SERVES 2

1 eating apple (I use
   Braeburn), thinly sliced
1 Tbsp sultanas (golden
   raisins)
juice of ½ lemon
pinch of brown sugar
   (or ½ tsp honey)
1 tsp ground cinnamon
a little butter or oil,
   for greasing the pan
2 tortilla wraps
1½ Tbsp almond butter
½ tsp chia seeds

TOP TIP

If you are cooking for 1, make the 2 servings and chill the remaining topping to add to porridge or yoghurt.

In a bowl, toss the apple slices and sultanas (golden raisins) with the lemon juice, sugar or honey and ½ teaspoon of the ground cinnamon.

Warm the butter or oil in a large frying pan (skillet) over a medium heat, add the apple mixture and cook for 8–10 minutes until softened.

Remove the apple mixture from the pan with a slotted spoon and set aside. Press a wrap into the bottom of the pan to heat through and allow to crisp up slightly. Remove and repeat with the second wrap.

To serve, spread the almond butter over the toasted wraps, top each with the apple mixture and sprinkle the chia seeds and remaining ½ teaspoon of cinnamon over the top.

Teff Pancakes

Teff is a grain from Ethiopia that many East African runners enjoy as a staple part of their diet. This tiny grain is naturally gluten-free and packed full of nutrients, including iron, calcium, magnesium and zinc, not to mention protein! Some runners have an increased risk of anaemia or have iron deficiencies, so using teff alongside more modern grains and flours can be a great way of boosting iron intake. Don't like bananas? No worries – use 250g (9oz/1 cup) unsweetened apple sauce instead.

SERVES 4

2 ripe bananas, peeled
1 egg, whisked
300ml (10fl oz/1¼ cups)
    milk or a milk alternative
2 tsp vanilla extract
230g (8oz/1¾ cups) teff flour
1 tsp baking powder
1 tsp ground cinnamon
    (optional)
vegetable or coconut oil,
    for frying

In a large bowl, thoroughly mash the bananas. Stir in the whisked egg, until combined, then stir in the milk and vanilla extract. Fold in the flour, baking powder and cinnamon, if using, until combined. The mixture should be quite a wet, spoonable consistency.

Heat about 1 teaspoon of oil in a large non-stick frying pan (skillet) over a medium heat add 1 large serving spoonful of batter into the pan. Fry for 2–3 minutes on one side until small bubbles appear, then gently flip and cook the other side for a further 2–3 minutes, until golden. Remove from the pan and set aside on a warm plate, or keep warm in a low oven. Repeat until all the batter has been used up, adding a little more oil to the pan each time it becomes dry. If your pan is big enough, feel free to cook more than one pancake at a time, ensuring that they are evenly spaced.

To serve, top with Greek yoghurt, fresh berries, maple syrup, honey, bacon, or your other favourite pancake toppings.

Any leftover pancakes can be frozen and reheated in the toaster for a quick week-day breakfast (you might need to toast them twice, depending on your toaster settings).

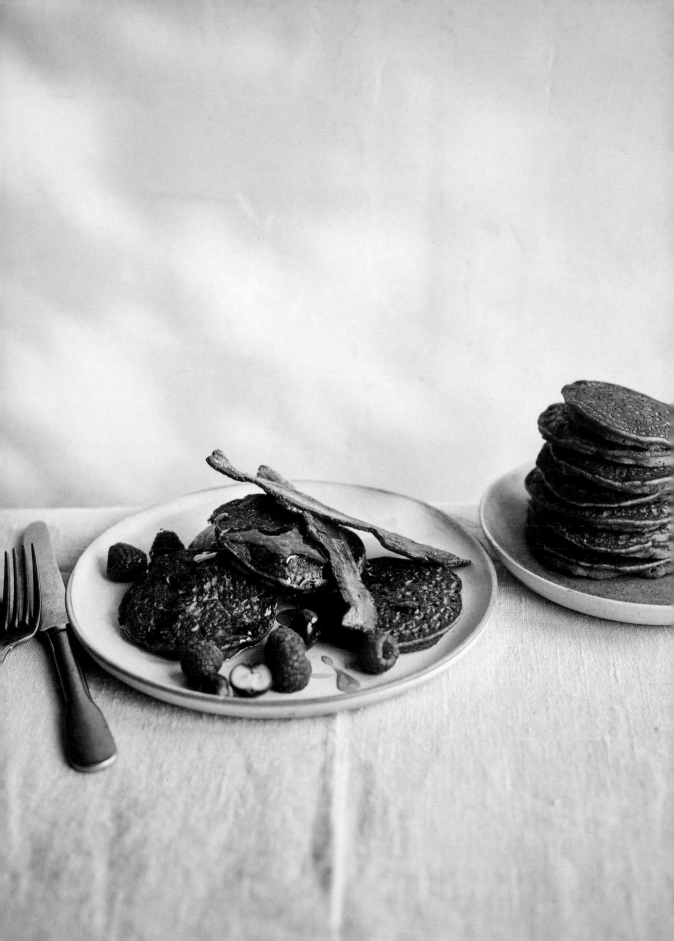

EAT LIKE AN ELITE

Sara & Ryan Hall's Teff Pancake

Sara and Ryan Hall are a running power couple and shared with me their favourite version of teff pancakes, using their preferred Muscle Milk protein powder (although feel free to sub in your favourite brand). According to Sara, 'It's packed with protein and essential nutrients to help fuel a morning workout or whatever else you need to tackle during the day. I like to top the pancake with a tablespoon of quality butter – it absolutely does not need syrup.'

Sara ran a marathon personal best at the Ottawa Marathon 2018, finishing in 2.26.20, and has the ninth-fastest US half marathon time, running a 1.09.27 in the Gold Coast Half in the same year. Ryan is the fastest American to run the Boston Marathon, finishing the 2011 race in 2.04.58, and represented the US in the 2008 and 2012 Olympics. He still holds the US half marathon record, running a 59.43 (the first American to break the one hour mark). He retired from professional running in 2016 and is now Sara's coach and the author of *Run the Mile You're In*.

SERVES 1–2
Depending on your post-run hunger!

70g (2½oz/½ cup) teff flour
3 Tbsp unsweetened cocoa powder
1 tsp baking powder
pinch Himalayan sea salt
1 scoop/portion (35g/1¼oz) chocolate protein powder
3 Tbsp Stevia
a little butter, for greasing the pan

In a large bowl or jug, mix together all the ingredients (except the butter), then slowly stir in enough water to achieve a batter of spoonable consistency.

Heat a little butter in a 25-cm (10-in) diameter non-stick frying pan (skillet) over a medium heat. Pour the batter into the pan and cook until air bubbles appear all over the surface of the pancake. Flip and cook for a further 20 seconds (if you like it gooey in the middle, like molten lava cake), then remove the pan from the heat. Otherwise, cook for longer, as desired.

"You can eat it directly out of the pan, if you like!" Sara Hall

Two-Ingredient Pancakes

Yep, these are literally just bananas and eggs. Although these pancakes can be made with only two ingredients, I tend to add quite a few more to the mix. Great additions are ground cinnamon, vanilla extract, ground ginger, or even blueberries, chopped nuts or chocolate chips! They are pretty sweet, so they don't need to be drowned in maple syrup. I serve mine with a dollop of Greek yoghurt and some fresh berries. I find these pancakes to be very light and so they make a great pre-run breakfast for those who find it hard to handle too much sitting in the stomach. They also provide protein, fat and carbs to keep up your energy!

SERVES 1

1 banana
2 eggs
cinnamon (optional)
vanilla (optional)
butter, for frying

TOP TIP

They can end up more like scrambled eggs if you're not careful. Make sure that your pan is non-stick and that you have a thin, wide spatula to flip your pancakes.

In a bowl, thoroughly mash the banana with a fork or potato masher until there are no large lumps left. Whisk in the eggs until fully combined.

Add any flavourings, such as cinnamon or vanilla, at this stage, if using.

Heat a little butter in a non-stick frying pan (skillet) over a medium-high heat until melted. These are easiest to cook as mini pancakes, so spoon in 2 tablespoons of mixture per pancake, making sure you leave plenty of space between each pancake. Cook for about 1 minute, or until the undersides are a golden brown and the edges have just started to set.

If you are adding any fruit, nuts or chocolate, add them to the wet batter just before flipping.

When it comes to flipping, do this slowly and carefully to avoid the pancakes breaking. Cook the other sides for about 1 minute, or until golden, before gently removing from the pan. Set aside on a warm plate or keep warm in a low oven. Repeat until all the batter has been used up.

You can cook the whole batch for a large breakfast, or save half for the following day – the batter will keep in the refrigerator for up to 3 days.

Overnight Oats

Overnight oats are one of my favourite weekday breakfasts – just mix up the night before and you're ready to go in the morning. Add your favourite toppings or whatever fruit you have – strawberries, mango, peaches and nectarines all work really well.

These oats are also perfect for those races where you don't have access to a kitchen to make your usual pre-race breakfast. Using a nut milk means they don't have to be stored in the refrigerator (although I do prefer them chilled). When I have these on a race morning, I swap the raspberries for a banana and add a good dollop of nut butter.

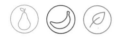

SERVES 1

40g (1½oz/scant ½ cup) quick-cook porridge oats (instant oatmeal)
1 tsp pumpkin seeds
2 Tbsp sultanas (golden raisins)
120ml (4fl oz/½ cup) unsweetened almond milk, plus extra if needed
40g (1½oz/scant ⅓ cup) raspberries

In a small bowl, Tupperware container or jar, combine the oats (oatmeal), pumpkin seeds, sultanas (golden raisins) and almond milk. Cover and chill in the refrigerator overnight, or for at least 6 hours.

The next day, or when ready to eat, top with raspberries and eat immediately.

TOP TIP

If you're making breakfast to eat on the go, you can mix it all together the night before. You can also make a large batch of the oats at the beginning of the week and mix up the toppings daily.

SUPERFOOD: OATS

Porridge (oatmeal) has had a resurgence as a cool, healthy breakfast option over the last few years, but the humble oat has been a staple in British diets for centuries. Packed with complex carbs, oats are broken down slowly, gradually releasing energy over a long period of time to keep your energy levels stable – perfect for endurance runners. Oats are also an often overlooked source of protein, which becomes a complete protein when mixed with dairy or a legume protein such as peanut butter. You'll find oats packed into plenty of the recipes in this book, not just breakfast options.

Not only are oats a great solution for replenishing glycogen stores, and a brilliant source of low-glycemic, soluble fibre, they also contain beta-glucan, a type of fibre that enhances the body's immune systems, helps stabilise appetite and may reduce levels of LDL cholesterol. They are also packed full of numerous minerals, including manganese, phosphorous, zinc, iron, magnesium and vitamin B1; not bad for a humble wholegrain.

In just half a cup of oats, you'll consume a third of your daily iron requirements – a nutrient that many runners are deficient in. Pair your oats with a source of vitamin C, such as berries, orange juice or baobab powder, to aid absorption.

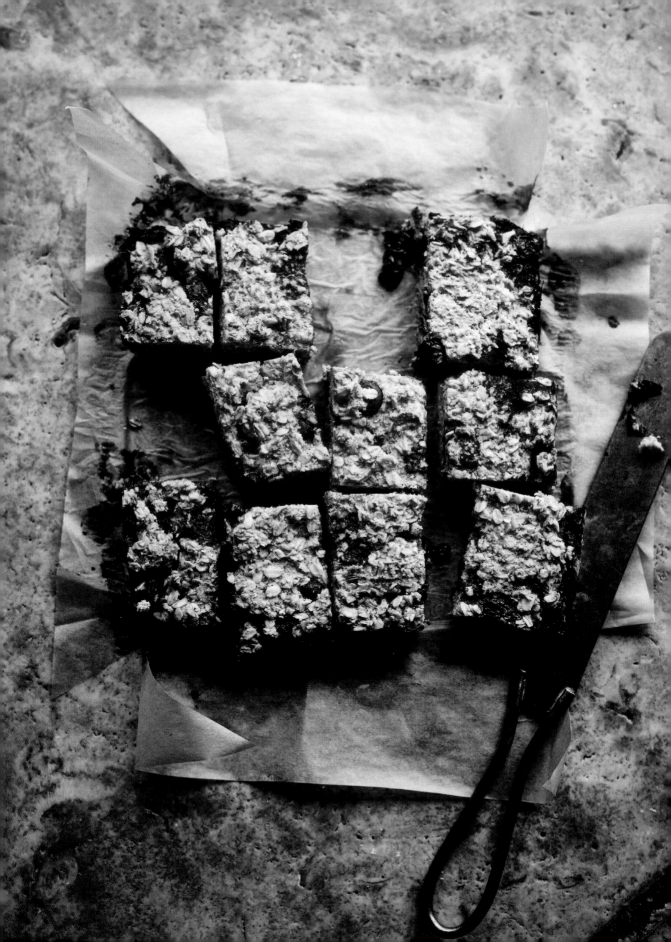

Oat Berry Breakfast Bars

Think you don't have time for breakfast? Think again. These breakfast bars can be made at the weekend and used throughout the week for a delicious brekkie to eat while on the go, during your commute or even at your desk. They also make a great afternoon snack. Refuel after a morning workout or prepare for one later in the day with these filling bars.

MAKES 12

250g (9oz/2⅔ cups) rolled (old-fashioned) porridge oats
1 large banana, thoroughly mashed
1 tsp vanilla extract
1 medium egg, whisked
220ml (7½fl oz/scant 1 cup) skimmed milk
2 Tbsp sunflower oil
1 tsp ground cinnamon
½ tsp baking powder
150g (5½oz/heaped 1 cup) raspberries
150g (5½oz/1¼ cups) blueberries

Preheat the oven to 180°C/350°F/gas mark 4 and line a 20-cm (8-in) square baking tin (pan) with baking paper.

Put 100g (3½oz/1 cup) of the oats into a food processor and process to a flour.

In a large bowl, mix together the banana, vanilla extract, egg, milk and oil until well combined. Stir in the oat flour and the remaining oats, cinnamon and baking powder, before folding in the berries.

Pour the batter into the prepared tin and bake for 35–40 minutes, or until the edges are golden and the mixture is set. Remove from the oven and let cool in the tin before slicing into 12 bars.

Wrap the bars in cling film (plastic wrap), store in the refrigerator and consume within 1 week. Alternatively, wrap each bar individually and freeze, then defrost overnight as needed.

Mediterranean Eggs

A nod of thanks goes to my friend Anna Sherriff, who whips up a version of this on every girls' weekend and summer holiday. It was particularly appreciated after parkrun on New Year's Day. This is something I prefer to eat after a run, rather than as pre-run fuel; however, if you're planning on running later in the day or have a late-start race, then just add a couple of pieces of toast to increase the carbohydrate intake and you should be good to go. This can also be upsized very easily to feed a large, hungry group.

SERVES 4

½ tsp olive oil
1 red onion, finely chopped
1 red (bell) pepper, deseeded and finely chopped
1 small courgette (zucchini), finely chopped
2 tomatoes, roughly chopped
8 medium eggs
30g (1oz/¼ cup) feta cheese, crumbled
small handful fresh coriander (cilantro) or flat-leaf parsley, chopped
salt and freshly ground black pepper, to taste
toast, to serve

Heat the olive oil in a large heavy pan over a low-medium heat, add the onion and red (bell) pepper and fry for 5 minutes. Add the courgette (zucchini) and tomatoes and cook, stirring occasionally, for a further 3 minutes.

Meanwhile, crack the eggs into a bowl, roughly whisk with a fork and season with salt and pepper. Pour the eggs into the pan and stir, using a wooden spoon to break up any lumps. Cook for a few minutes until nicely scrambled, making sure you keep the mixture moving as much as possible.

Once the eggs are cooked to your liking, quickly remove from the pan to prevent overcooking and serve immediately, sprinkled with feta and chopped coriander (cilantro) or parsley, with toast on the side.

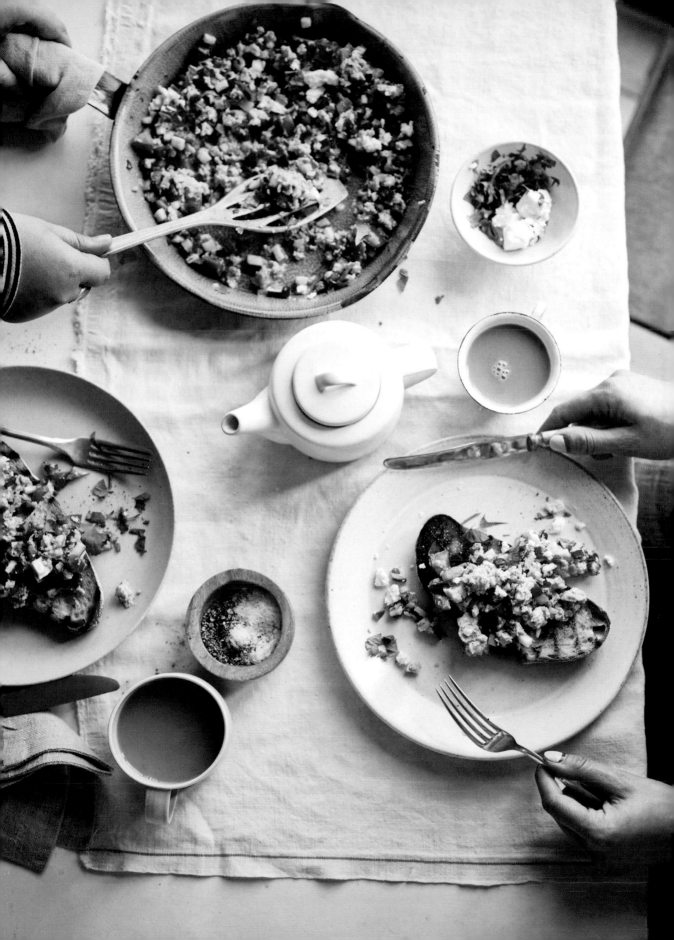

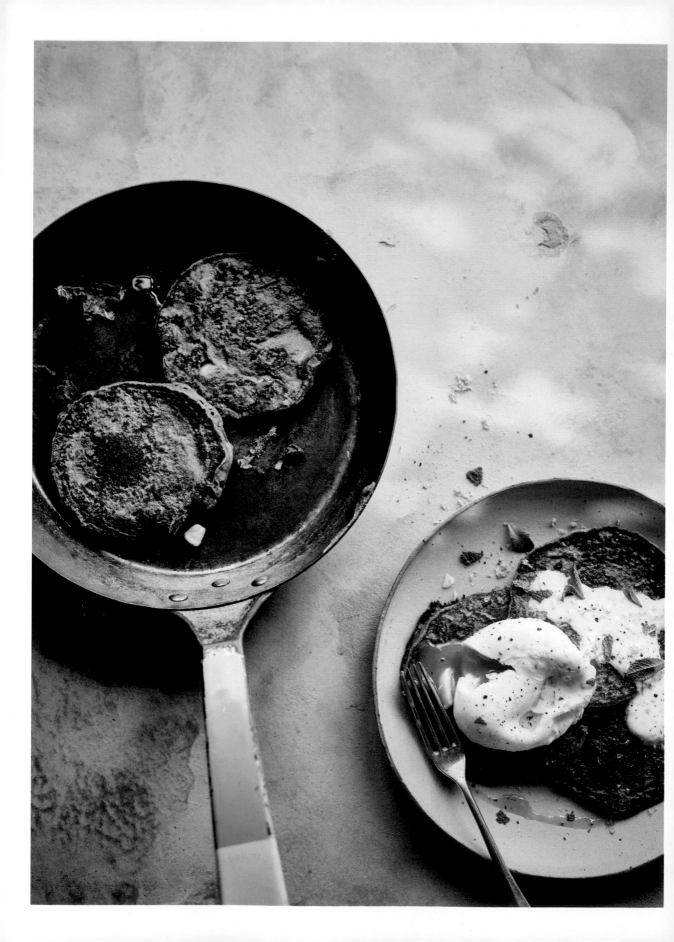

Broccoli and Sweetcorn Fritters

These brilliantly green fritters are packed with veg and make a delicious post-run brunch or a quick and nutritious weeknight dinner. I tested this recipe on the kids that I nanny and they suggested that these be included in the book.

SERVES 4

1 x 340-g (12-oz) can sweetcorn (corn), drained
200g (7oz) long-stem broccoli
150g (5½oz) baby spinach
1 small red onion, finely chopped
175g (6oz/1⅓ cups) self-raising flour
6 large eggs (if using)
250g (9oz/generous 1 cup) full-fat Greek yoghurt, or dairy-free alternative
1 Tbsp vegetable oil
finely grated zest and juice of 1 lemon
small handful fresh mint, finely chopped
salt and freshly ground black pepper, to taste

Preheat the oven to 150°C/300°F/gas mark 2.

Reserve about 40g (1½oz/generous ⅓ cup) of the sweetcorn (corn) and set aside. Place the remaining corn in a powerful blender or food processor and blitz, then add the broccoli, spinach, onion, flour, 2 of the eggs, 3 tablespoons of the yoghurt and plenty of seasoning. Process until smooth, scraping down the sides from time to time, to ensure it is well combined. Stir in the reserved corn.

Heat a little of the oil in a large non-stick frying pan (skillet) over a medium-high heat. Dollop 2 tablespoons of the batter into the pan and spread out slightly until about the size of your palm. Repeat to make 2 more fritters, leaving space between them. Cook for 2–3 minutes until the fritters begin to turn golden around the edges, then carefully flip with a wide spatula and cook on the other side until golden, 2–3 minutes.

Keep the fritters warm in the oven while you repeat with the remaining batter to make 12 fritters in total, adding a little more oil as necessary if the pan seems dry.

Meanwhile, bring a large, deep saucepan of water to a simmer. Crack an egg into a ramekin or coffee cup, then pour it into the simmering water. Working quickly, add the remaining 3 eggs in the same way. Poach for 4 minutes or until the whites feel firm but the yolks are still soft. Lift the eggs out with a slotted spoon and drain on paper towels.

In a small bowl, mix together the remaining yoghurt with the lemon zest and juice, and stir in the chopped mint.

Serve 3 fritters per person, each topped with a poached egg and a dollop of the yoghurt sauce.

Savoury Quinoa Porridge

I know the idea of savoury porridge (that's oatmeal to non-Brits) might seem a little strange, but it's actually delicious and perfect for those who prefer to save the sweet stuff until later in the day. I use quinoa flakes for added protein, but feel free to use jumbo or quick-cook oats (whatever you have at home) and adjust the cooking times accordingly. I think it tastes a little bit like grits (or the grits that I tried on a recent trip to Savannah, anyway!). Stir in a little grated cheese while cooking, if you like. For vegans, omit the egg and scatter over a handful of toasted pumpkin seeds. Pictured opposite, with Porridge with Blueberry Chia Jam (see page 66).

SERVES 1

50g (2oz/scant ½ cup)
   quinoa flakes
240ml (8fl oz/1 cup) milk
   or unsweetened dairy-
   free milk of choice
1 Tbsp soy sauce
1 tsp olive or avocado oil,
   plus extra if needed
1 small clove garlic, crushed
50g (2oz) mushrooms,
   finely chopped
1 spring onion (scallion),
   finely sliced
1 egg (if using)
salt and freshly ground
   black pepper, to taste
¼ avocado, sliced, to serve
chilli sauce, to serve
   (optional)

In a small saucepan over a low-medium heat, combine the quinoa flakes and milk and cook for 8–10 minutes, or until the milk is absorbed and the quinoa is soft, stirring regularly. Stir in the soy sauce and season to taste.

Meanwhile, heat the oil in a small frying pan (skillet) over a high heat and fry the garlic for 1 minute, then add the mushrooms and cook for 5–7 minutes until softened. Stir in the spring onion (scallion) and fry for 1 minute, then carefully lift out the vegetables with a slotted spoon and set aside.

Crack the egg into the same pan, adding a little extra oil if the pan looks too dry, and fry for 3 minutes, or until the white is set and the yolk is soft

Spoon the quinoa porridge into a bowl and top with the mushroom mixture, avocado slices and fried egg. Serve with chilli sauce, if you like.

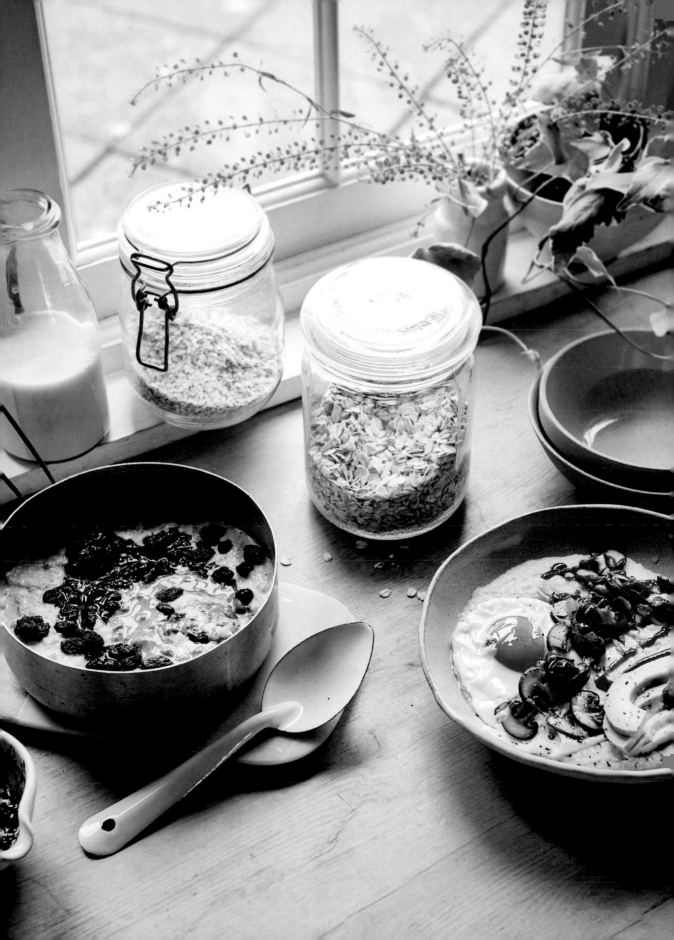

Porridge with Blueberry Chia Jam

Throughout the winter, porridge is my staple breakfast. Both during the week and at weekends, I like to make a warming bowl whenever I have the time. I don't have a microwave, so I've perfected the art of stovetop (OK, induction top) porridge, while making coffee and packing my lunch at the same time. My top tip is to add the dried fruit while cooking the oats – this plumps up the fruit and makes it far juicier. I also like to use jumbo rolled (old-fashioned) oats for texture, but feel free to use quick-cook oats to speed things up. A number of runners struggle with eating dairy before a run (or try to limit their intake), so using a dairy-free milk or water in this pre-run porridge is perfect. In my opinion, unsweetened oat or almond milk tastes best, but use whichever you prefer. (Pictured on page 65, left.)

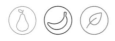

SERVES 1

For the blueberry chia jam (makes 8 servings):
150g (5½oz/¾ cup) frozen blueberries
1 Tbsp chia seeds

For the porridge:
50g (2oz/½ cup) jumbo rolled (old-fashioned) oats
240ml (8fl oz/1 cup) oat milk or other dairy-free milk, plus extra as needed
2 Tbsp raisins or sultanas (golden raisins)
1 tsp almond butter or other nut butter, to serve

To make the jam, heat the frozen berries in a small saucepan over a low heat until they thaw and become juicy, about 10 minutes. Using a fork or potato masher, mash the berries until most have broken down, then stir in the chia seeds. Simmer gently for about 3 minutes, then remove the pan from the heat.

Allow the jam to cool and thicken for 10 minutes. Enjoy immediately with your porridge or chill in the refrigerator for up to a week.

To make the porridge, combine the oats, milk and dried fruit in a small saucepan and place over a low-medium heat. Cook for 5–7 minutes, stirring regularly, until the milk has been absorbed and the oats are soft. Add a little extra milk if it looks dry.

Serve immediately, topped with the nut butter and a dollop of the blueberry chia jam.

Chocolate Peanut Butter Granola

I have my friend Emma and Purely Elizabeth's chocolate peanut butter granola to blame for this recipe. I would come back from trips to America with suitcases stuffed with bags of granola, and once, in Phoenix, I took a cab for 20 minutes to Target just to buy granola to take home. I had to come up with a cheaper solution – making my own chocolate granola rather than having to fly to the US (or pay any more excess baggage fees!).

This is another recipe that improves with age. It will keep in an airtight container for up to 3 months and is perfect with berries and yoghurt as a post-run breakfast or evening dessert.

MAKES 12 SERVINGS

250g (9oz/2⅔ cups) jumbo rolled (old-fashioned) oats
70g (2½oz/¾ cup) mixed nuts, roughly chopped (I use pecans and walnuts)
70g (2½oz/⅓ cup) peanut butter (no added sugar)
100g (3½oz/⅓ cup) maple syrup
1 tsp vanilla extract
70g (2½oz/⅓ cup) coconut oil
3 Tbsp cocoa powder
1 tsp ground cinnamon
pinch sea salt (optional)

Preheat the oven to 160°C/325°F/gas mark 3. Grease and line a large baking sheet with baking paper.

Spread the oats and nuts in a single layer over the prepared baking sheet and bake for 10 minutes.

In a large saucepan, melt together the peanut butter, maple syrup, vanilla extract and coconut oil. Stir in the toasted oats and nuts, along with the cocoa and cinnamon and mix together until well combined.

Pour the mixture back onto the prepared baking sheet and bake for 25–30 minutes until the mixture has formed into clumps. Sprinkle over the salt, if using. Allow to cool completely on the baking sheet before transferring to an airtight container.

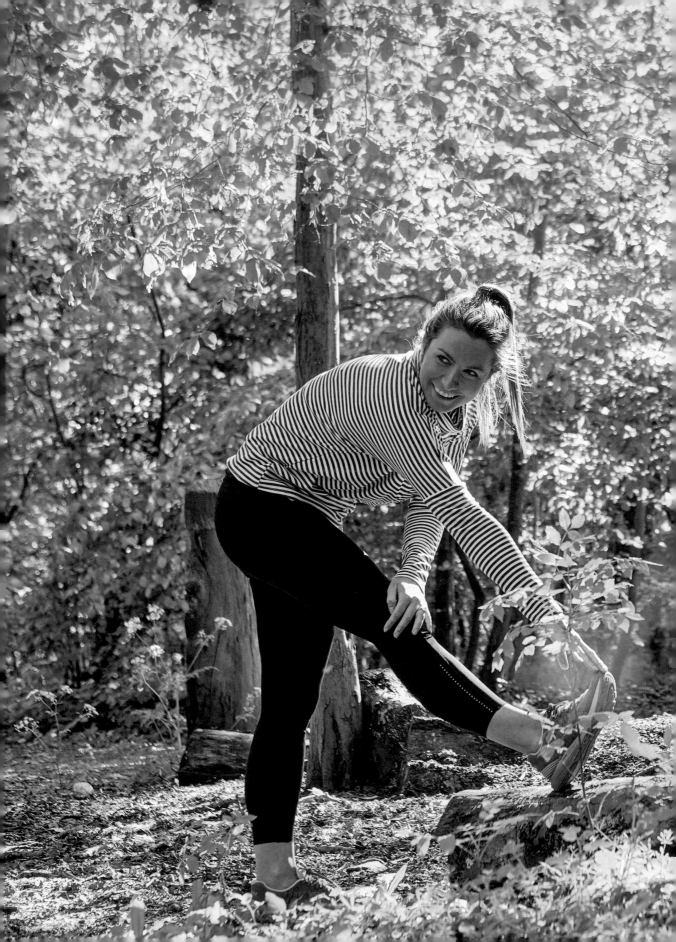

20–MINUTE MEALS

I prefer to get my runs done in the morning. If I leave it until the afternoon, I find that life, work, exhaustion and excuses can come into play. However, while on my dietetic hospital placements, I got into the habit of running home from work a couple of days a week or fitting an evening class into my schedule, meaning I often didn't get home until past 8 o'clock. When it's late, you just want to be able to make something fast and easy, but you also want it to be nutritious so that you can refuel post-exercise (or prepare yourself for the following day's run). These meals are on the table within 20 minutes (and there's no shame if you cook and eat them in your sports kit!).

When it comes to speeding up your evening cooking, my advice is to plan your meals ahead if possible, so that you can double-up on ingredients (rather than having a refrigerator full of half-eaten tubs or packets) and avoid that HANGRY supermarket shop. Buying time-saving ingredients (whether that's pre-cut veg, microwavable rice, canned beans and pulses, or pre-cooked meat and fish) can be a great way to shave down cooking time, but still enable you to prepare healthy, mid-week meals.

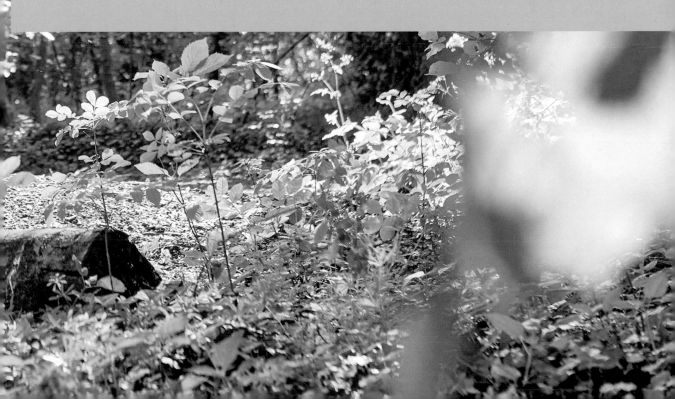

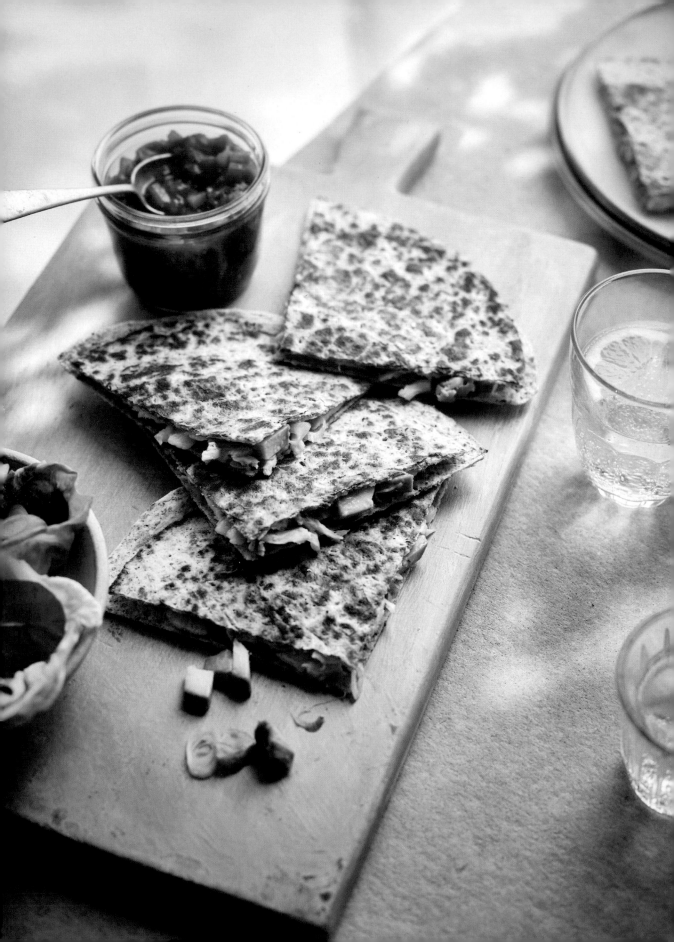

Chicken and Avocado Quesadillas

You might have noticed a theme with these quick meals – a lot of them are Mexican-inspired. I think that Mexican is my favourite style of food (okay, maybe it's more Tex-Mex). I just need to actually visit Mexico now, to try the real deal! This recipe is inspired by my *Good Housekeeping* colleague Monaz's quesadilla recipe.

SERVES 2

1 cooked chicken breast (about 125g/4½oz), roughly chopped
1 avocado, finely chopped
3 spring onions (scallions), finely sliced
few dashes Tabasco sauce
50g (2oz) mixed lettuce leaves
4 large tortillas (I use seeded tortillas, but any will work)
50g (2oz/generous ½ cup) Cheddar cheese, coarsely grated (shredded)
salt and freshly ground black pepper, to taste
tomato salsa (store-bought), to serve

Preheat the oven to its lowest setting.

In a large bowl, mix the chicken with half of the avocado and spring onions (scallions). Mix in the Tabasco sauce and add some seasoning, to taste. Set aside.

Make a salad with the remaining avocado and spring onion and the lettuce and set aside.

Heat a large non-stick frying pan (skillet) or griddle pan over a medium heat. Lay a tortilla in the pan and top with a quarter of the cheese and allow it to melt slighty. Spoon over half of the chicken mixture then sprinkle over another quarter of the cheese and press a second tortilla on top. Cook for 3–5 minutes, then flip the quesadilla (this is best done by sliding it onto a plate, topping it with another plate or board, inverting it, then sliding it back into the pan). Cook for a further 3–5 minutes on the other side, or until slightly golden and crispy.

Transfer the cooked quesadilla to a baking sheet and place in the warm oven, while you make the second quesadilla in the same way.

Serve with the salad and a tablespoon of tomato salsa on the side of each one.

Middle-Eastern Turkey Burgers

Making your own burgers may sound time-consuming, but it doesn't need to be. Using a food processor means that they come together in no time. You can use diced chicken in place of turkey, if you prefer. Or swap out the burger buns and wrap the patties in iceberg lettuce for a crunchy gluten-free option.

SERVES 4

400g (14oz) turkey breast
1 x 400-g (14-oz) can
    chickpeas (garbanzo
    beans), drained
small handful fresh coriander
    (cilantro)
1½ tsp harissa paste
1 tsp za'atar spice mix
    (see tip)
1 Tbsp vegetable oil

To serve:
4 wholewheat bread rolls
    or burger buns
1 large tomato, cut into
    4 slices
large handful salad leaves
3 Tbsp tzatziki (optional)

In a food processor, pulse the turkey until coarsely minced (ground). Add the chickpeas (garbanzo beans), coriander (cilantro), harissa paste and za'atar and pulse until well combined. Shape the mixture into 4 equal-sized patties.

Heat the oil in a large frying pan (skillet) over a medium-high heat. Add the burgers and fry for 8 minutes on each side until golden brown and cooked through.

Meanwhile, slice the bread rolls or burger buns horizontally and lightly toast. Fill each with a burger, a slice of tomato and some lettuce. Serve with tzatziki and extra salad leaves, if you like.

TOP TIP

If you don't have any za'atar spice mix, you can make your own by combining 1 teaspoon ground cumin, 1 teaspoon ground sumac, 1 teaspoon ground coriander, 1 teaspoon dried thyme or oregano, and 1 teaspoon sesame seeds. Store in an airtight container.

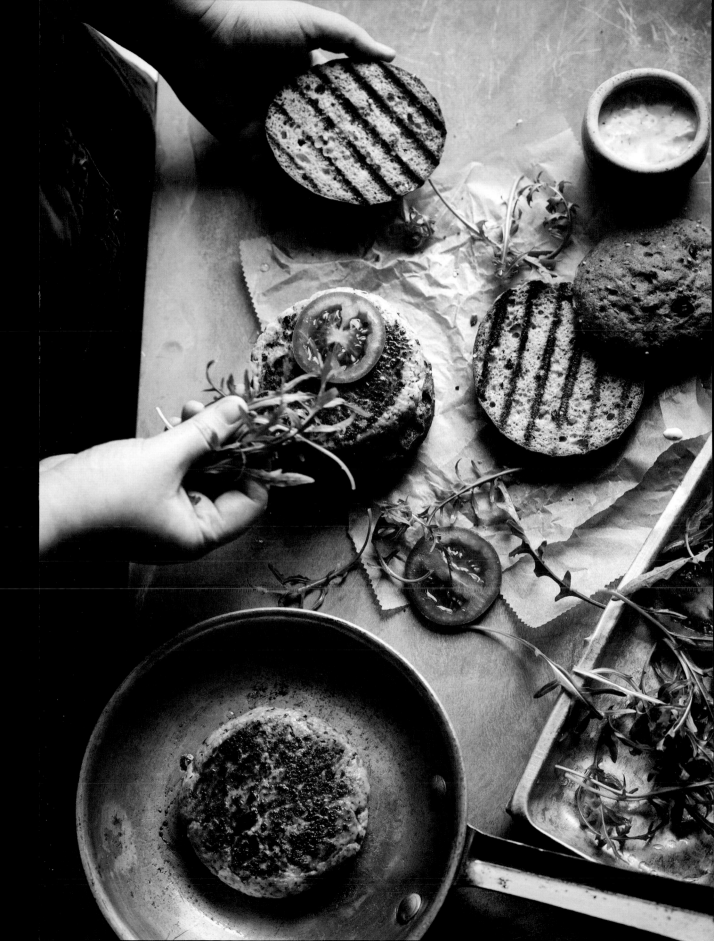

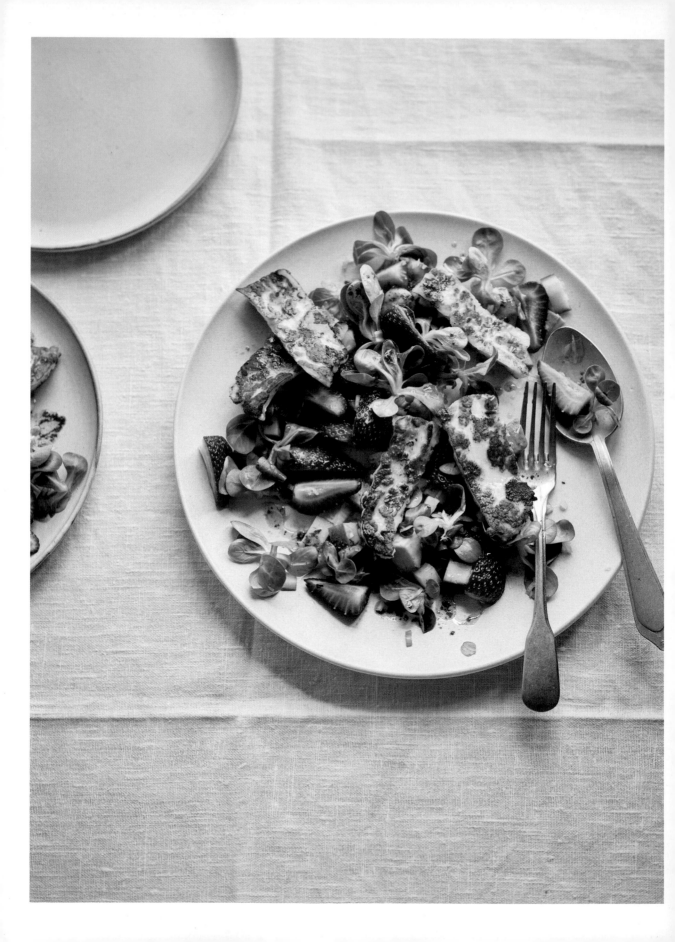

Strawberry and Halloumi Salad

A friend's mum introduced me to strawberries in salad 15 years ago, and so began an everlasting obsession with fruit in savoury dishes. You'll see quite a few recipes with the combination dotted throughout the book. Fruit adds a fresh twist and natural sweetness, and counts towards your five-a-day!

SERVES 2

1 tsp vegetable oil
250g (9oz) halloumi, cut
    into slices 1cm (½in) thick
½ cucumber, chopped
100g (3½oz) lamb's lettuce
1 avocado, roughly chopped
200g (7oz/2 cups)
    strawberries, hulled
    and quartered
2 spring onions (scallions),
    finely chopped

For the dressing:
3 Tbsp olive oil
1 Tbsp balsamic vinegar
small handful fresh basil
    leaves
salt and freshly ground black
    pepper, to taste

Heat the oil in a large non-stick frying pan (skillet) over a medium heat, add the halloumi and carefully fry for a few minutes on each side until golden, turning occasionally.

Meanwhile, combine the cucumber and lettuce in a large bowl. Add the avocado, strawberries and spring onions (scallions) and toss through.

In a food processor or blender, blitz together the dressing ingredients and season to taste.

Divide the salad among 4 plates, top with the hot halloumi and drizzle with the dressing.

Cheat's Paella

This is one of those dishes where you can use up whatever veg, meat or fish you have in the refrigerator or freezer and it tastes great. I think it's excellent with leftover roast chicken and king prawns (jumbo shrimp), but it also works with squid, roast pork, chorizo, white fish, or even just packed full of vegetables, as here.

SERVES 4

1 tsp olive oil
1 onion, finely sliced
2 red, orange or yellow (bell) peppers, deseeded and finely sliced
1 clove garlic, crushed
2 tsp smoked paprika
pinch saffron
150g (5½oz/1 cup) cherry tomatoes, halved
300g (10½oz/1½ cups) orzo pasta
750ml (25fl oz/3¼ cups) vegetable (or chicken or fish stock) (bouillon)
100g (3½oz/¾ cup) frozen peas
large handful fresh flat-leaf parsley, roughly chopped
salt and freshly ground black pepper, to taste
lemon wedges, to serve

Heat the oil in a large frying pan (skillet) or paella pan (with a lid) over a medium heat, add the onion and peppers and gently fry for 8 minutes, until softened. Add the garlic, paprika, saffron and tomatoes and cook for 1 minute, then add the orzo pasta, stock (bouillon) and peas. Bring to the boil, then reduce to a simmer, cover with the lid, and cook for 10 minutes, stirring occasionally. Season to taste, then stir through the parsley.

Serve with lemon wedges.

SUPERFOOD: TOMATOES

The trusty tomato comes in many shapes, sizes and varieties. They are a good source of vitamin C, potassium, folate, and vitamin K, which has a positive effect on bone mineral density and decreases fracture risk.

Cooking tomatoes actually increases the amount of lycopene (a powerful antioxidant that can decrease the risk of bone density loss) available to our bodies. This nutrient is fat-soluble, meaning that eating it alongside healthy fats, such as olive oil, eggs and avocado, increases absorption.

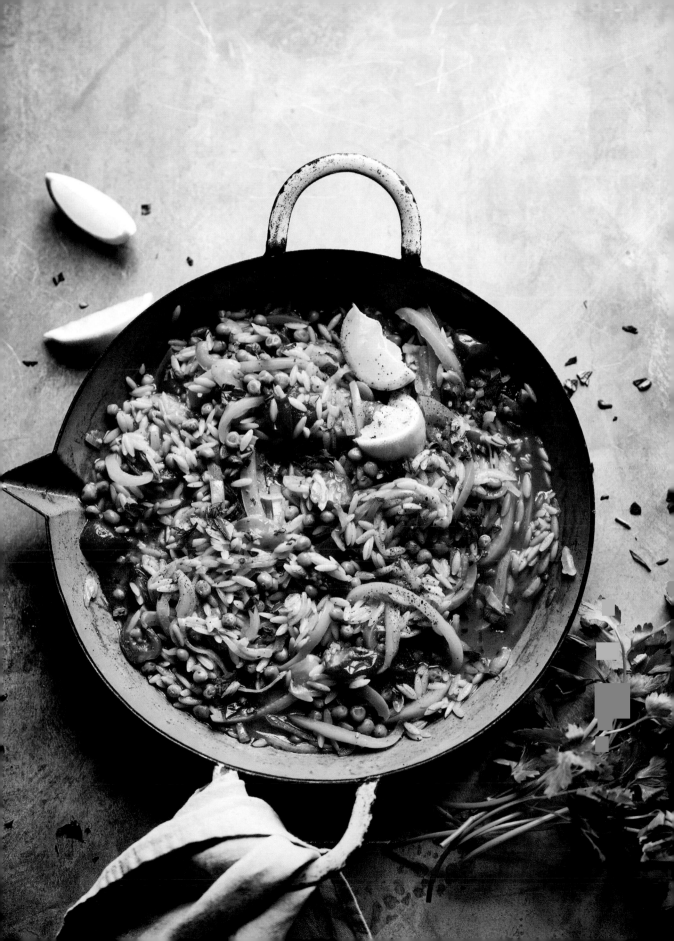

Tomato Poached Eggs

Eggs make the perfect quick-cook dinner, providing plenty of protein per serving. The kids I nanny call this dish 'Everything in the Fridge Eggs', as I usually throw in whatever veggies, cheese, meat or beans are on hand.

SERVES 2–3
Depending on your
post-run hunger!

1 tsp olive oil
1 onion, finely chopped
1 red (bell) pepper, deseeded
   and roughly chopped
2 cloves garlic, crushed
1 tsp dried chilli (red pepper)
   flakes
1 Tbsp tomato purée (paste)
2 x 400-g (14-oz) cans
   chopped tomatoes
1 Tbsp balsamic vinegar
1 x 400-g (14-oz) can butter
   (lima) beans (borlotti
   beans, black beans or
   chickpeas/garbanzo beans
   will also work), drained
50g (2oz) baby spinach
4 medium eggs
salt and freshly ground black
   pepper, to taste

To serve:
30g (1oz/¼ cup) feta cheese,
   crumbled
large handful flat-leaf parsley,
   roughly chopped
toasted sourdough slices or
   pita breads

Warm the oil in a large sauté pan (with a lid) over a low-medium heat, add the onion and (bell) pepper and gently cook, stirring, for 8 minutes until they begin to soften. Add the garlic and dried chilli (red pepper) flakes and cook for 1 minute, before adding the tomato purée (paste), chopped tomatoes and balsamic vinegar. Bring to the boil, then reduce the heat and simmer until slightly thickened. Stir in the beans and spinach and allow the spinach to wilt slightly, then season to taste.

Use a wooden spoon to make 4 small holes in the sauce and crack an egg into each one. Cover the pan with the lid and simmer for a further 8 minutes, or until the egg whites are cooked but the yolks are still runny.

Serve, garnished with the crumbled feta and chopped parsley, with toasted sourdough or pita breads on the side.

Beef and Broccoli Stir-Fry

To make this taste even better, leave your beef to marinate
while you go for your run or gym workout!

SERVES 2

250g (9oz) sirloin steak,
  thinly sliced
4 Tbsp low-sodium soy sauce
1½ Tbsp plain (all-purpose)
  flour
175ml (6fl oz/¾ cup)
  low-sodium stock
  (bouillon), chicken, beef
  or vegetable will work
2 Tbsp sweet chilli sauce
1 Tbsp rice wine vinegar
1 clove garlic, crushed
1-cm (½-in) piece fresh root
  ginger, peeled and finely
  grated (shredded)
½ tsp dried chilli (red pepper)
  flakes
1 large head broccoli, cut into
  small florets
1 tsp sesame or vegetable oil
2 spring onions (scallions),
  finely sliced
1 x 250-g (9-oz) packet
  microwave rice, to serve
small handful peanuts, finely
  chopped, to garnish

Put the steak in a large bowl with 2 tablespoons of the soy sauce and 1 tablespoon of the flour. Cover and chill while you cook the rest of the recipe or ideally leave it to marinate for longer, but no longer than 8 hours.

In a jug, mix together the stock (bouillon), sweet chilli sauce, vinegar, garlic, ginger, dried chilli (red pepper) flakes and remaining 4 tablespoons soy sauce. Whisk in the remaining ½ tablespoon flour and set aside.

Heat a large sauté pan or wok over a high heat and add 5 tablespoons of water. Immediately thow in the broccoli and stir-fry for 3–4 mins, until al dente. Remove the broccoli and set aside.

Return the pan to the heat and add the oil, then add the marinated steak and stir-fry until just cooked through. Remove the steak from the pan and set aside with the broccoli.

Pour the stock mixture into the pan and bring to the boil, then reduce to a simmer and cook for about 3 minutes until slightly thickened. Stir in the steak and broccoli, along with most of the spring onions (scallions).

Meanwhile, cook the rice according to the packet instructions.

Serve the stir-fry over a portion of rice, garnished with the remaining spring onions and the peanuts.

Sprout Satay

Having actively avoided Brussels sprouts at Christmas for over 25 years, I have now become a little bit obsessed. The difference between boiled, overcooked sprouts and sweet roasted sprouts is vast. However, if you're not a fan (even after trying them lovingly roasted), you can swap them for broccoli or cauliflower.

SERVES 2

250g (9oz) Brussels sprouts, trimmed and halved
1 Tbsp coconut oil, melted
1 clove garlic, crushed
1-cm (½-in) piece fresh root ginger, finely grated (minced)
200g (7oz) baby sweetcorn (baby corn), roughly chopped
200g (7oz) mange tout (snow peas)
2 Tbsp korma/medium curry paste
2 Tbsp chunky peanut butter
200ml (7fl oz/scant 1 cup) full-fat coconut milk
soy sauce, to taste
1 lemon: ½ for juicing; ½ cut into 2 wedges
2 spring onions (scallions), finely sliced
salt and freshly ground black pepper, to taste
brown rice or noodles, to serve

Preheat the oven to 200°C/400°F/gas mark 6.

Arrange the sprouts in a roasting pan in a single layer and drizzle over half of the coconut oil. Season with salt and pepper and roast for 15 minutes until soft and golden.

Meanwhile, heat the remaining coconut oil in a large non-stick sauté pan, add the garlic and ginger and fry for 1 minute, then add the baby sweetcorn (baby corn) and fry for a further 3 minutes. Add the mange tout (snow peas) and fry for a further 2 minutes, then remove the vegetables from the pan and set aside.

Add the curry paste and peanut butter to the pan, along with 100ml (3½fl oz/scant ½ cup) water, and mix together. Stir in the coconut milk and allow the mixture to bubble and reduce slightly. Add the cooked vegetables back to the pan and season to taste. Add a drizzle of soy sauce, squeeze over the juice of the lemon half and sprinkle over the spring onions (scallions).

Serve the satay with brown rice or noodles, with lemon wedges on the side.

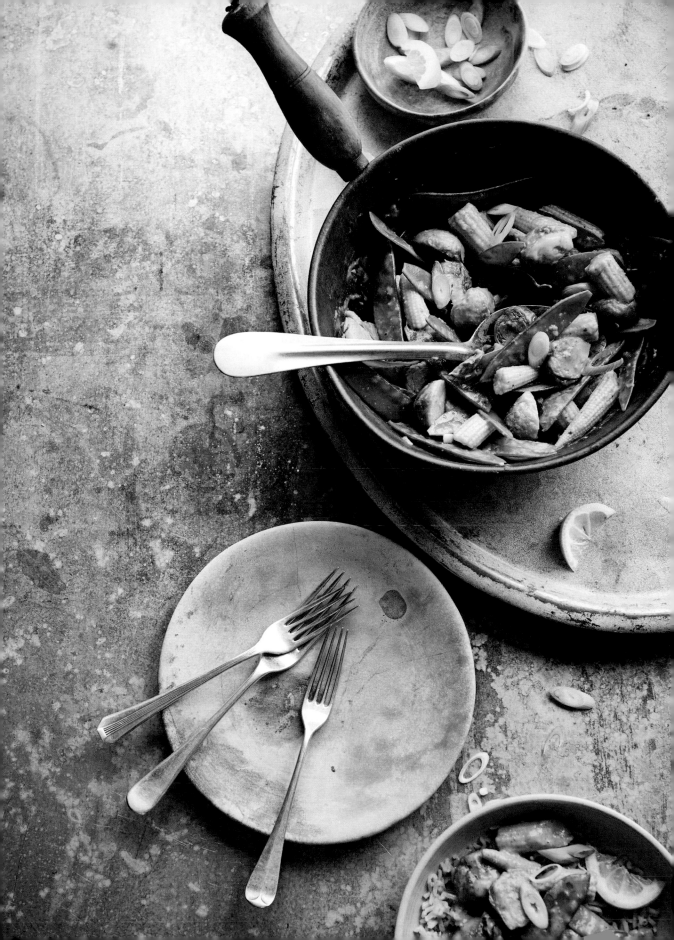

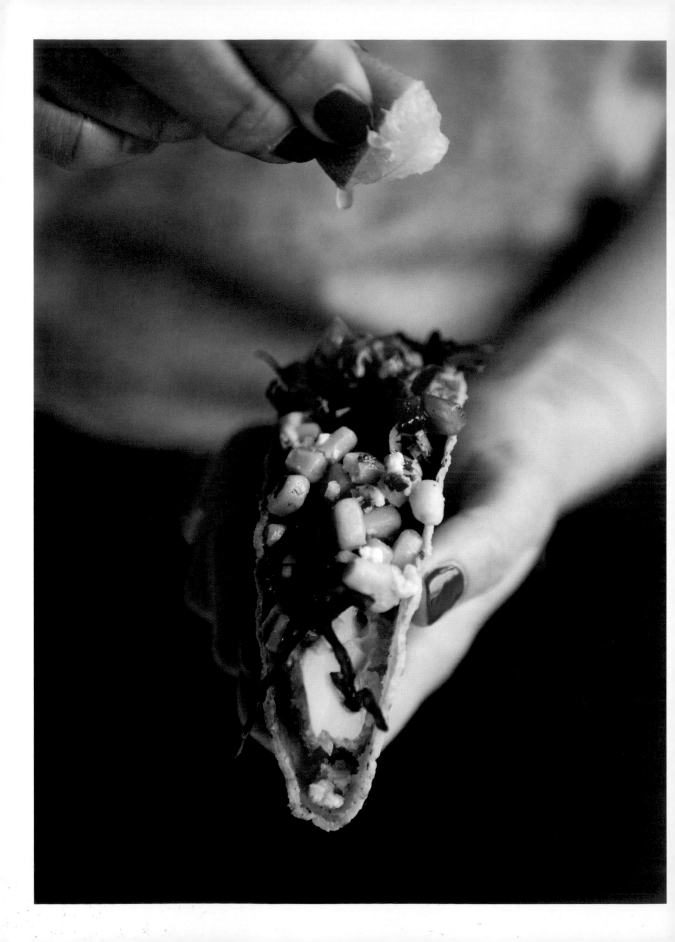

Fast Fish Tacos

I've mentioned it before, but I'm obsessed with Mexican food. On a trip to Portland with my Mum, I had the best fish tacos in a neighbourhood restaurant. While these aren't quite authentic *tacos de pescado*, they are pretty tasty! You can substitute the fish for breaded or grilled chicken or prawns (shrimp). Vegetarians can omit the fish and mix in a can of black beans with the sweetcorn for added protein.

SERVES 4

2 breaded cod fillets (about 350g/12½oz)
1 Tbsp butter
1 x 200-g (7-oz) can unsalted sweetcorn (corn), drained
1 red chilli, finely chopped
30g (1oz/¼ cup) feta cheese
200g (7oz) tomatoes, finely chopped
1 red onion, finely chopped
large handful fresh coriander (cilantro), finely chopped
1 tsp extra virgin olive oil
juice of 1 lime, plus extra lime wedges to serve
¼ red cabbage, finely shredded
8–12 taco shells or tortillas
salt and freshly ground black pepper, to taste

Preheat the oven to 200°C/400°F/gas mark 6.

Place the breaded cod on a baking sheet and bake for 15 minutes or according to the packet instructions.

Meanwhile, heat the butter in a large saucepan over a low-medium heat, add the sweetcorn (corn), and cook for 3–5 minutes, stirring, until heated through. Add the black beans, if using. Season with salt and pepper, then stir through half of the chilli and all of the feta. Remove from the heat and place in a serving bowl.

In a small bowl, mix together the tomatoes with half of the onion and most of the coriander (cilantro), reserving a little for garnish. Mix in the olive oil and half of the lime juice. Season to taste.

In a separate bowl, toss the cabbage together with the remaining onion and chilli and squeeze over the remaining lime juice.

Warm the tacos or tortillas in the oven for the final 2 minutes of the fish's cooking time.

Remove the baked fish from the oven, cut into thin slices and place in another serving bowl.

Serve all the bowls and the tacos or tortillas, along with some extra lime wedges and the reserved fresh coriander, for people to help themselves. Any leftovers make a great packed lunch!

Mexican Bean Salad

This salad is a veggie twist on one of my favourite salads of all time, created by my old boss and mentor, Meike Beck. I am so grateful to her for everything she taught me about cooking, life, work and gin drinking! Add cooked chicken or prawns (shrimp) if you want some extra protein.

SERVES 4

2 heads of gem lettuce, shredded
200g (7oz) cherry tomatoes, halved
1 avocado, finely chopped
1 x 400-g (14-oz) can kidney beans, drained and rinsed
1 x 400-g (14-oz) can black beans, drained and rinsed
1 x 200-g (7-oz) can unsalted sweetcorn (corn), drained and rinsed
2 spring onions (scallions), finely sliced
30g (1oz/¼ cup) Cheddar cheese, coarsely grated (shredded)
3 Tbsp sour cream
3 Tbsp lime juice
pinch freshly ground black pepper
4 small handfuls tortilla chips (Meike and I like the Cool Original Doritos)

In a large bowl, mix together the lettuce, tomatoes and avocado. Toss through the beans and sweetcorn (corn), then stir in the spring onions (scallions) and cheese.

In a small bowl, mix together the sour cream and lime juice with a pinch of black pepper, then pour over the salad and toss to combine.

Divide among 4 plates, and crunch a small handful of tortilla chips over each salad.

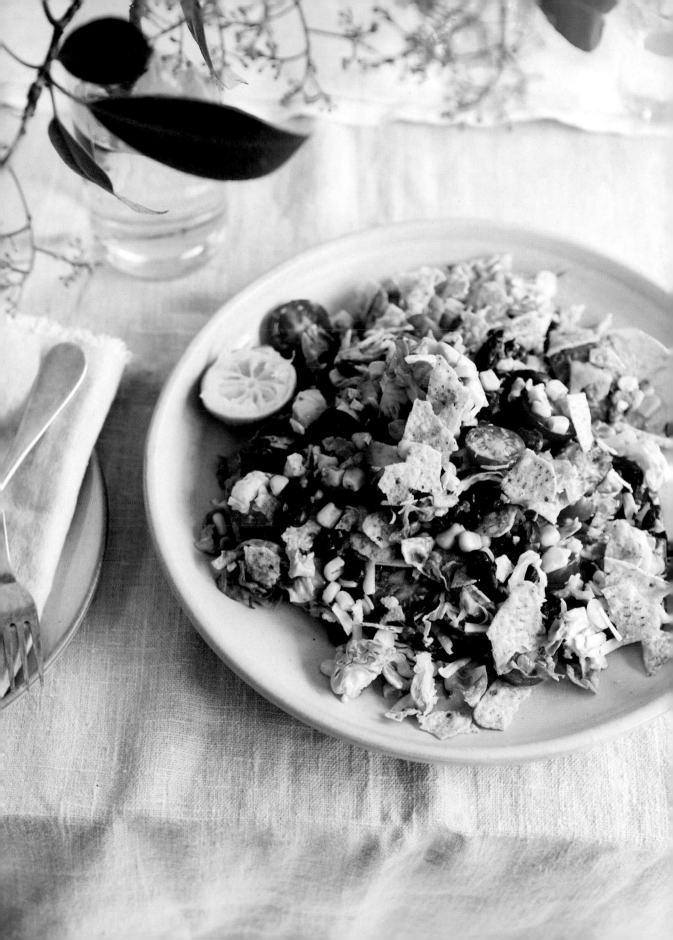

Prawn and Pineapple Fajitas

This dish would also work well with white fish, salmon or chicken. For a vegan option, replace the shellfish with a 400-g (14-oz) can of drained kidney beans or black beans and use a dairy-free yoghurt.

SERVES 4

1 Tbsp olive or vegetable oil
1 red onion, finely sliced
2 (bell) peppers (I use green and orange), deseeded and sliced
1 clove garlic, crushed
1-cm (½-in) piece fresh root ginger, peeled and finely grated
1 Tbsp fajita spice mix (see tip)
300g (10½oz) raw king prawns (jumbo shrimp)
100g (3½oz) fresh or canned pineapple, chopped into 2.5-cm (1-in) cubes
large handful fresh coriander (cilantro), chopped
juice of 1 lime, plus extra to taste
8 flour or corn tortillas
1 ripe avocado, cut into slices 1cm (½in) thick
full-fat natural (plain) yoghurt
salt and freshly ground black pepper, to taste

Preheat the oven to 160°C/325°F/gas mark 3.

Heat the oil in a large sauté pan over a low heat, add the onion and peppers and gently fry for 10 minutes, until softened. Add the garlic and fry for another 1 minute. Stir in the ginger and fajita spice mix, then add the prawns (shrimp) and cook for 5 minutes, stirring, until pink and cooked through. Add the pineapple and half of the coriander (cilantro), gently heat through, then squeeze over the lime juice and season to taste.

Meanwhile, put the tortilla wraps in the oven to warm through.

Divide the filling among the tortilla wraps and top each with a few avocado slices, a sprinkling of coriander and a dollop of yoghurt, before rolling up. Serve immediately.

TOP TIP

You can buy a fajita spice mix in most supermarkets; to make your own, mix together 1 teaspoon paprika, ½ teaspoon cayenne pepper, 1 teaspoon ground cumin and ½ teaspoon ground ginger. Store the leftover mix in an airtight container.

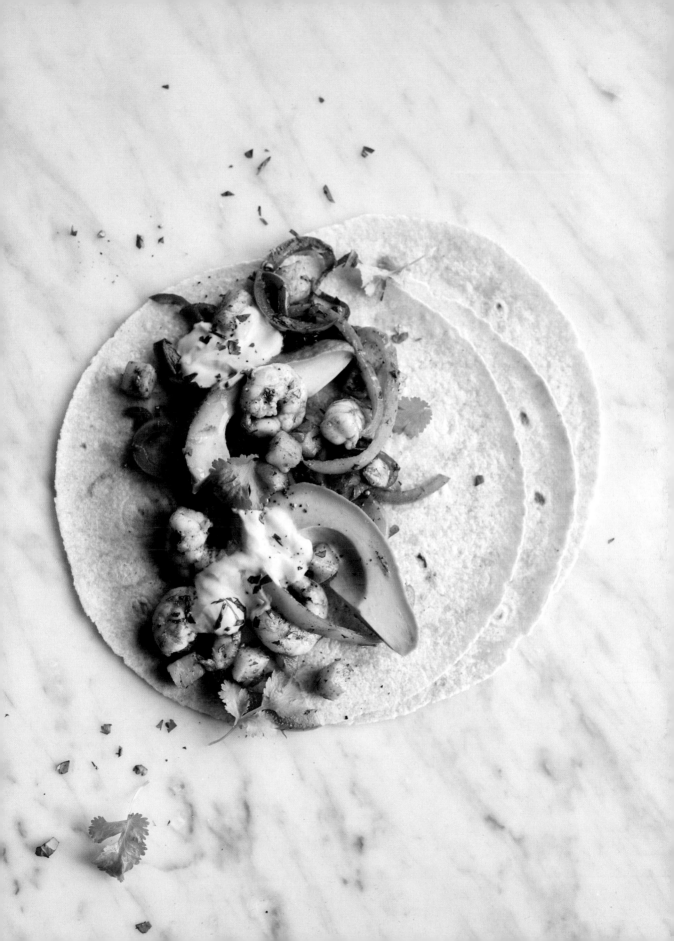

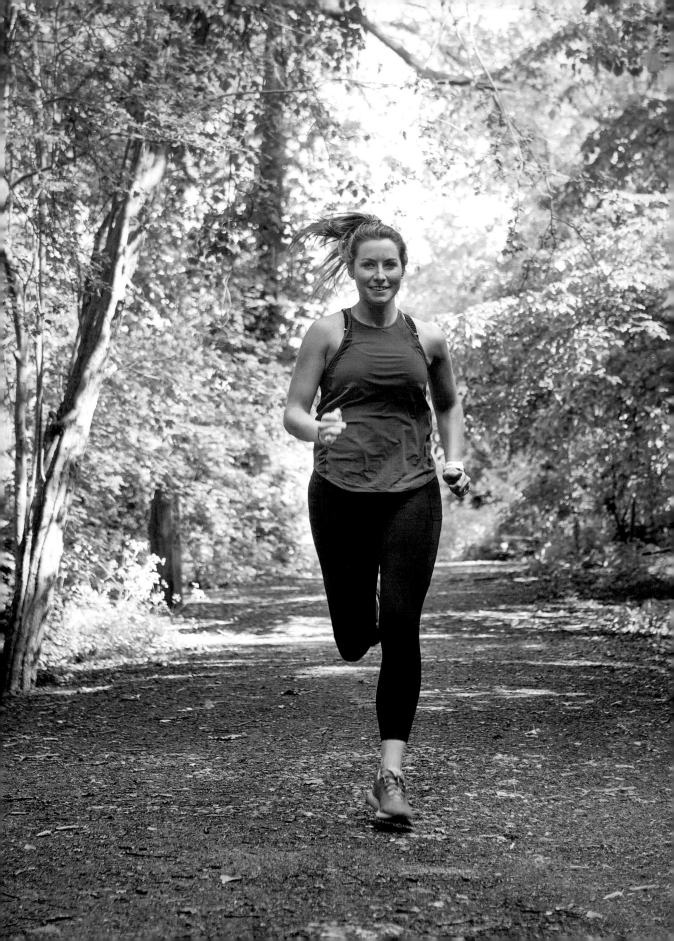

PRE-RUN FUEL

I took a poll on Instagram to find out what other runners ate before a race or long run. Runners are a pretty superstitious bunch and many stick to their tried and true 'night-before' meal religiously, even when travelling. Pizza, lasagne and pasta with tomato sauce came out as favourites, so instead of re-inventing the wheel, I've included some delicious homemade versions of these.

There are also some new recipes that I hope will become firm faves. The Balinese Beetroot Curry (page 95) with mild spices that won't upset your stomach, plenty of carbs from the chickpeas (garbanzo beans) and rice, plus the endurance-boosting power of beetroot (beets – see also page 156), has become a regular dish in my house. Another dish I really love is the Avocado Carbonara (page 90) – dairy-free and refreshingly light, this is a great pre-race dish or weeknight supper, and is particularly good eaten in the summer, preferably al fresco with a glass of rosé wine.

In the lead-up to a race, you'll want to gradually increase your carbohydrate intake (although often the term 'carb-loading' is taken to the extreme!) to optimize your energy stores. Increasing your carb intake for 2–3 days pre-race, combined with tapering (reducing your training load), will help ensure your muscle glycogen levels are topped up and ready to race.

To avoid feeling sluggish, I try to stick to normal portion sizes and have an extra snack or two in the days prior to a race. Alternatively, adding a sports drink or smoothie can be a great way to increase your carb intake without feeling 'stuffed'.

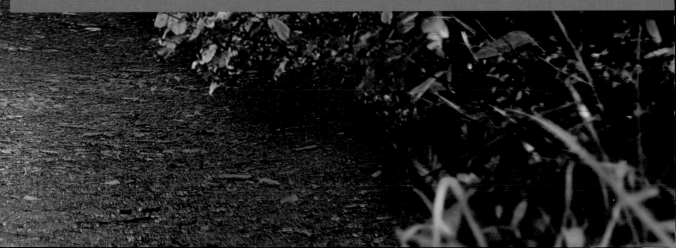

Avocado Carbonara

I love carbonara. However, before a race I try to avoid anything too heavy, so came up with this creamy option instead. It's a great alternative for those who try to avoid dairy the night before a long run. Not only is this great pre-race, but it also makes a speedy weeknight dinner. If you want to make it veggie or vegan-friendly, simply swap the pancetta for peas and use vegan cheese. Save any leftovers for a lovely cold pasta salad.

SERVES 4

400g (14oz) spaghetti
50g (2oz) pancetta, roughly
   chopped
1 very ripe avocado
juice of 1 lemon
handful fresh basil
250ml (8½fl oz/generous
   1 cup) almond milk
150g (5½oz) cherry tomatoes,
   roughly chopped
30g (1oz/scant ½ cup)
   Parmesan or other hard
   cheese, grated, plus extra
   to serve

Bring a large saucepan of water to the boil and cook the pasta according to the packet instructions.

Meanwhile, heat a large dry frying pan (skillet) over a high heat and fry the pancetta for 4–5 minutes until brown and crispy. Remove from the heat and set aside.

In a food processor or high-powered blender, combine the avocado, lemon juice, basil and almond milk and blitz until smooth.

Drain the pasta, reserving a little of the cooking water, and return it to the pan. Stir through the avocado sauce, some of the reserved pasta water (if needed) and the chopped tomatoes, crisp pancetta and grated cheese. Serve immediately, garnished with extra cheese.

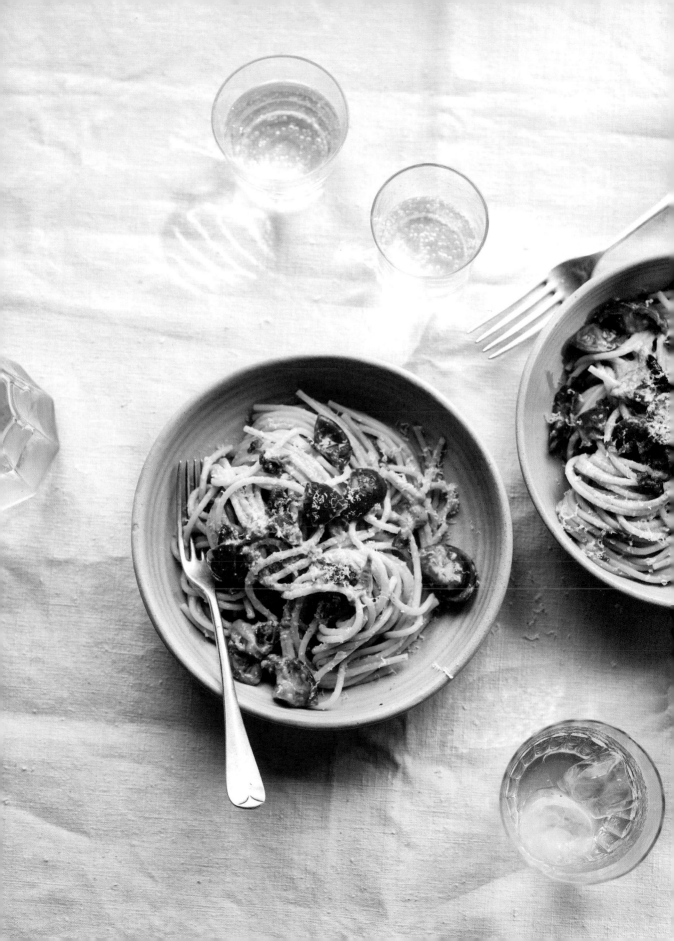

Beetroot and Goat's Cheese Pasta

What's the best type of pasta to eat? Wholegrain? White? Lentil pasta? Personally, I eat mostly wholegrain, except the night before a long run or race when I want to reduce my fibre intake (and don't need the extra protein). If you're eating this pre-run, then I'd suggest opting for the white refined version; however, the rest of the time, choose the pasta you like most. There are some amazing edamame and lentil options available, which have a higher protein and fibre content than traditional dried pasta. I prefer wholegrain for the taste and nutritional profile. But pasta should be enjoyed ... so eat the one you like (and just measure out the appropriate portion).

SERVES 4

250g (9oz) cooked beetroot (beets), roughly chopped
2 red onions, roughly chopped
1 Tbsp olive oil
400g (14oz) pasta of choice
3 Tbsp roughly chopped pecans
100g (3½oz/scant ½ cup) soft goat's cheese
salt and freshly ground black pepper, to taste

Preheat the oven to 180°C/350°F/gas mark 4.

Arrange the beetroot (beets) and onions in a single layer in a roasting pan, drizzle with the oil and season with salt and pepper. Roast for 15 minutes.

Meanwhile, bring a large saucepan of water to the boil and cook the pasta according to the packet instructions.

Carefully remove the roasted vegetables from the roasting pan and set aside. Scatter the pecans over the same pan and return to the oven to toast for 5 minutes.

Meanwhile, put most of the roasted beetroot (reserve a little for garnish), all of the roasted onion and three-quarters of the goat's cheese into a food processor and blitz until smooth. Season to taste.

Drain the pasta and remove the toasted pecans from the oven. Toss the beetroot sauce through the pasta and divide among four serving bowls. Serve immediately, garnished with the reserved beetroot, remaining goat's cheese and toasted pecans.

Sweet Potato Gnocchi

I've kept this really simple with just butter and sage, but I suggest serving it with garlic-roasted broccoli or steamed long-stem broccoli. Prefer a tomato sauce for your gnocchi? Serve it with the tomato pizza sauce (page 98) instead of the butter and sage. This also makes a great starter for six at a dinner party. To make it in advance, boil the gnocchi but do not fry, then sauté at the last minute to ensure that they are piping hot and golden before serving.

SERVES 4, OR 6 AS A STARTER

500g (1lb 2oz) sweet potatoes
100g (3½oz/scant ½ cup) ricotta cheese
50g (2oz/scant ¼ cup) thick full-fat Greek yoghurt
200g (7oz/1½ cups) plain (all-purpose) flour, plus extra for dusting
drizzle olive oil
30g (1oz/2 Tbsp) butter
small handful fresh sage leaves
salt and freshly ground black pepper, to taste
30g (1oz/scant ½ cup) grated Parmesan cheese, to serve

Preheat the oven to 200°C/400°F/gas mark 6.

Roast the sweet potatoes for about 1 hour until soft (alternatively cook for 7 minutes on high in the microwave). Halve and scoop the flesh out of the skins and transfer to a bowl.

Mash the potato flesh together with the ricotta and yoghurt and plenty of salt and pepper. Stir in the flour, about a quarter at a time, and try to avoid over-mixing. Once the dough becomes thicker and easier to handle, transfer to a clean, floured work surface. Bring the dough together into a loaf-like shape (about 9 x 23cm/3½ x 9in) and cut slices off the short side. Stretch and roll each slice out into a long thin snake, before cutting into smaller pieces, each about 2.5cm/1in long.

Meanwhile, bring a large pan of water to the boil. Add the gnocchi to the pan in batches to avoid overcrowding. They are cooked when they start to float, about 5 minutes. Carefully remove from the pan with a slotted spoon to a waiting bowl and toss in a little olive oil to stop them sticking together.

When all the gnocchi have been cooked, melt the butter in a large frying pan (skillet) over a medium-high heat. Add the gnocchi and fry for 10 minutes, then add the sage leaves and fry for another 5 minutes, until the sage is crispy and the gnocchi are golden.

Serve the gnocchi and crispy sage leaves sprinkled with grated Parmesan.

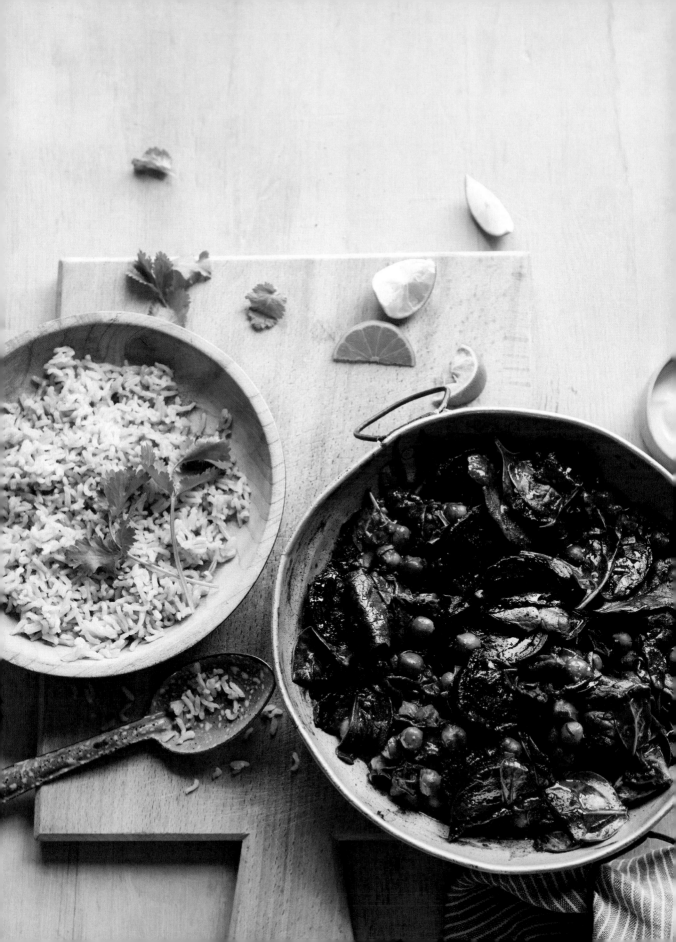

Balinese Beetroot Curry

Okay, bear with me on this one... I was very sceptical when the Mum for whom I nanny asked me to make this – and even more sceptical when I was given a slightly bare-bones recipe to work from. But, you know what, it worked. The sweetness from the beetroot goes really well with the warm spices; in fact, the curry is even more delicious the next day when the spices have developed.

SERVES 4

500g (1lb 2oz) raw beetroot (beets), peeled and cut into thin wedges
2 tsp olive oil
2 tsp ground cumin
2 tsp caraway seeds
1 tsp ground turmeric
30g (1oz/⅓ cup) cashews
1½ tsp linseeds
1 onion, finely sliced
2 cloves garlic, crushed
2.5-cm (1-in) piece fresh root ginger, peeled and finely chopped
1 red chilli, deseeded and finely chopped
large handful fresh coriander (cilantro), leaves picked stalks finely chopped
1 x 400-ml (14-fl oz) can coconut milk
1 x 400-g (14-oz) can chickpeas (garbanzo beans), drained
300g (10½oz) baby spinach
juice of 1 lime
salt and freshly ground black pepper, to taste
cooked brown rice, to serve

Preheat the oven to 180°C/350°F/gas mark 4.

Put the beetroot (beet) wedges into a roasting pan and drizzle with half of the olive oil. Roast for 30 minutes.

Meanwhile, put the spices, cashews and linseeds into a high-powered food processor or spice grinder and blitz together.

Heat the remaining olive oil in a large saucepan over a medium heat, add the onion and fry for 10 minutes until soft. Add the garlic, ginger, chilli and the spice mixture, and fry for a further 2 minutes. Add the chopped coriander (cilantro) stalks and the coconut milk and bring to a simmer. Finally, add the roasted beetroot, chickpeas (garbanzo beans) and spinach and cook for a further 5 minutes until the spinach has wilted and chickpeas are heated through.

Squeeze in the lime juice, garnish with the coriander (cilantro) leaves and season to taste and serve with brown rice.

Winter Salad

I hate having cold salads for lunch during the winter; instead, I opt for soups and reheated dinner leftovers. However, this warm salad bridges the gap, providing warmth (and a kick of heat) during those dark months. It's also great in summer when the saltiness of the cheese pairs perfectly with a glass of rosé. I've used Greek Kefalotyri cheese, but this works really well with halloumi, goat's cheese or feta, too.

SERVES 4

750g (1lb 10oz) butternut squash, peeled, deseeded and cut into 2.5-cm (1-in) cubes
2 red onions, each cut into 8 wedges
1 Tbsp olive oil
1 vegetable stock (bouillon) cube
300g (10½oz/scant 2 cups) pearled spelt
200g (7oz) cavolo nero or kale
1 red chilli, deseeded and finely sliced
200g (7oz) Greek Kefalotyri cheese
plain (all-purpose) flour, for dusting
salt and freshly ground black pepper, to taste

For the dressing:
2 Tbsp olive oil
juice of ½ lemon
½ tsp runny honey
1 small clove garlic, crushed

Preheat the oven to 200°C/400°F/gas mark 6. Line a large roasting pan with baking paper.

Toss the squash and red onion with ½ tablespoon of the olive oil and put into the prepared pan. Season with salt and pepper and roast for 20 minutes.

Meanwhile, bring a large saucepan of water to the boil, add the stock (bouillon) cube and stir to dissolve. Add the spelt and reduce to a simmer, then cook for 25–30 minutes until the spelt is tender but still a little chewy.

Add the cavolo nero or kale to the vegetables in the roasting pan and return to the oven to roast for a further 5–7 minutes, or until the greens are starting to crisp up.

Drain the spelt and add it to the roasting pan along with the chilli and roast for a final 5 minutes.

Run the cheese briefly under cold running water, then toss it in a little flour to coat.

Heat the remaining ½ tablespoon of olive oil in a large frying pan (skillet) over a medium heat. Add the cheese to the pan and fry for 5 minutes, or until golden and slightly melted. Remove from the pan and cut into long strips, about 2.5cm (1in) wide.

Mix together the dressing ingredients and season to taste.

Serve the roasted salad while still warm, topped with the cheese slices and with the dressing drizzled over.

Cajun Chicken Pasta

Make sure to use full-fat cream cheese for this recipe, otherwise it could split when heated. If you only have half- or low-fat, ensure that you remove the pan from the heat before stirring it through. Trust me on this – I once had to wash and strain our dinner before starting again with the sauce! Feel free to use prawns (shrimp) or a vegetarian alternative in place of chicken, if you prefer.

SERVES 4

2 chicken breasts
1 tsp cayenne pepper
2 tsp smoked paprika
2 tsp ground cumin
1 Tbsp olive oil
400g (14oz) pasta of choice
150g (5½oz/generous 1 cup) frozen peas
1 red onion, finely sliced
2 red (bell) peppers, deseeded and finely sliced
2 large tomatoes, roughly chopped
1 chicken stock (bouillon) cube
100g (3½oz/scant ½ cup) full-fat cream cheese
salt and freshly ground black pepper, to taste

Preheat the oven to 200°C/400°F/gas mark 6.

Loosely wrap the chicken breasts in cling film (plastic wrap), place on a work surface and bash with a rolling pin until flattened, then unwrap. Stir together the spices, then sprinkle over both sides of the chicken breasts.

Heat the oil in a large frying pan (skillet) over a medium heat, add the chicken breasts and sear on both sides, then use a slotted spoon to lift out the chicken and transfer to a baking sheet. Bake in the oven for 10 minutes, until cooked through.

Bring a large saucepan of water to the boil and cook the pasta according to the packet instructions. When the pasta has 5 minutes' cooking time left, add the peas to the water. Drain, reserving 500ml (17fl oz/generous 2 cups) of the cooking water, and set aside.

Meanwhile, add the onion and (bell) peppers to the same frying pan and fry for 5 minutes, then add the tomatoes and cook for 5 minutes until softened.

Stir the stock (bouillon) cube and cream cheese into the reserved pasta cooking water, then stir this into the pepper mixture. Bring to the boil and cook until reduced and slightly thickened. Stir in the pasta and peas and season to taste.

Divide the pasta among 4 bowls, carefully slice the chicken and serve on top of the pasta.

Pre-Run Pizza

Runners love pizza. Perfect either for pre-run fuelling or as a post-race celebratory dinner, this homemade version is delicious. I love pepperoni or ham and pineapple on my pizza – I know that is sacrilege for Italians, but on the photoshoot for this book we found that the whole team loved it, so I can't be that weird! The tomato sauce makes double what you will need to top the pizzas, but it can be frozen or kept in the refrigerator for up to a week.

MAKES 2 X 25-CM (10-IN) PIZZAS

For the dough:
230g (8oz/1⅔ cups) strong white (bread) flour, plus extra for dusting
½ tsp salt
½ tsp fast-action dried yeast
2 Tbsp extra virgin olive oil, plus extra for greasing
150ml (5fl oz/⅔ cup) lukewarm water

For the sauce:
2 cloves garlic, crushed
1 x 400-g (14-oz) can chopped tomatoes
small handful fresh basil leaves
pinch sugar (optional)
1 tsp balsamic vinegar

For the toppings:
1 x 125-g (4½-oz) buffalo mozzarella ball, drained and torn into pieces
handful of your choice of ham, cooked chicken, pineapple chunks, cooked mushrooms
freshly ground black pepper

To make the dough, sift the flour and salt into a large mixing bowl, then stir in the yeast. Make a well in the middle of the mixture, then pour in the oil and water, stirring until you have a soft but not sticky dough.

Turn the dough out onto a lightly floured work surface and knead for 10 minutes until smooth and elastic. Put into a lightly oiled bowl, cover with a clean tea (dish) towel and place in a warm place to rise for 1 hour.

Meanwhile, make the pizza sauce. Put the garlic, tomatoes, most of the basil, sugar (if using) and balsamic vinegar into a food processor and blitz together until smooth. Set aside.

Preheat the oven to 230°C/450°F/gas mark 8 and lightly grease 2 large baking sheets.

Knock the air out of the dough and divide it in half. On a lightly floured surface, use a rolling pin to roll out each half to a circle 25cm (10in) in diameter, then transfer to the prepared baking sheets.

Spread the bases with enough pizza sauce to cover, then top with mozzarella and your preferred toppings. Bake for 10–15 minutes, or until crisp and golden.

Serve, garnished with the remaining basil leaves and plenty of freshly ground black pepper.

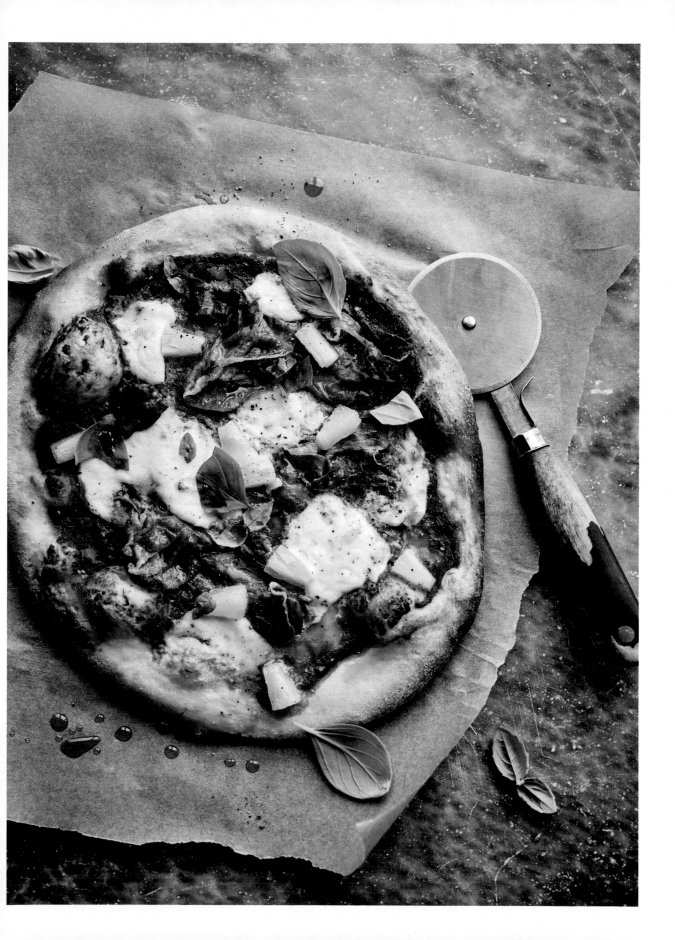

EAT LIKE AN ELITE

Kathrine Switzer's Pre-Race Prawn Pasta

I had the pleasure of meeting Kathrine Switzer at a talk she gave at the Boston Marathon in 2017. She was running the race 50 years on from her first Boston event. Back then, women weren't oficially allowed to enter; however, thanks to a helpful coach and boyfriend, Kathrine was able to run with a bib, proving to everyone that women were not 'too fragile' to run 26.2 miles. Kathrine went on to win the New York City Marathon in 1974 and was at one stage ranked the sixth-fastest woman in the world over the distance. Her famous Boston bib number, 261, has since been retired from the race and is now the name of her charity, '261 Fearless', which aims to empower and unite women through running.

SERVES 4

1 Tbsp olive oil
1 onion, finely chopped
6 tomatoes, roughly chopped
1 clove garlic, crushed
1 courgette (zucchini), coarsely grated
½–1 red chilli, finely chopped (optional)
400g (14oz) spaghetti
350g (12½oz) cooked king prawns (jumbo shrimp)
large handful fresh basil, finely chopped, plus extra whole leaves to serve
salt and freshly ground black pepper, to taste
30g (1oz/scant ½ cup) Parmesan cheese, finely grated, to serve

Heat the oil in a large frying pan (skillet) over a medium heat, add the onion and tomatoes and cook for 10 minutes, stirring, until softened and the tomatoes have broken down (you can mash them with the back of the spoon to help them along). Stir in the garlic, courgette (zucchini) and chilli (if using) and cook for a further 2 minutes.

Meanwhile, bring a large saucepan of water to the boil and cook the pasta according to the packet instructions.

Stir the cooked prawns (shrimp) and chopped basil into the tomato sauce and season to taste.

Drain the pasta, reserving a little of the cooking water, then mix the pasta into the sauce, adding a little of the pasta water to loosen if necessary.

Serve, garnished with basil leaves and Parmesan.

TOP TIP

Kathrine told me that she would avoid eating chilli the night before a marathon, so keep that in mind if you have a sensitive stomach.

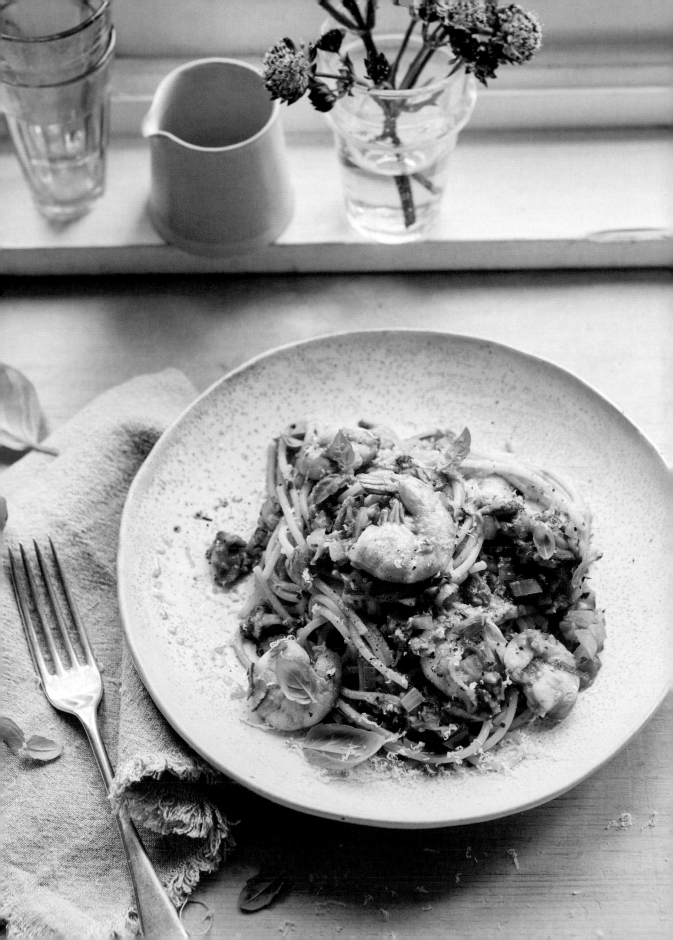

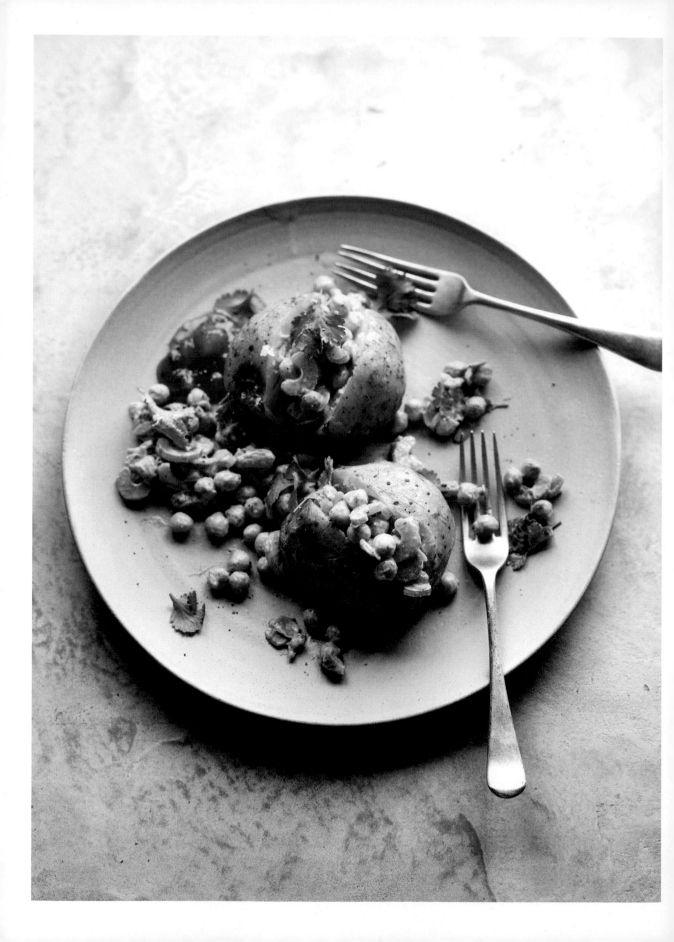

Coronation Chickpea Salad

Coronation chicken is a British dish created in 1953 for Queen Elizabeth II's coronation luncheon. Traditionally, it is made with young roasting chickens, wine, a bouquet garni, apricot purée and a creamy curry sauce. This version swaps the chicken for chickpeas (garbanzo beans) and uses mango chutney and apricots for sweetness, and celery for a crunch. It takes a lot less time to make than the original dish. For Americans, this is like a curried chicken salad, only using chickpeas, and much lighter than usual.

SERVES 4–6

2 Tbsp mild curry paste
2 x 400-g (14-oz) cans
   chickpeas (garbanzo
   beans), drained and rinsed
2 Tbsp light mayonnaise,
   or dairy-free alternative
100g (3½oz/scant ½ cup)
   full-fat Greek yoghurt,
   or dairy-free alternative
1 Tbsp mango chutney
2 stalks celery, finely chopped
50g (2oz/⅓ cup) dried
   apricots, finely chopped
50g (2oz/¾ cup) flaked
   (slivered) almonds,
   toasted if you like
large handful fresh coriander
   (cilantro)
salt and freshly ground black
   pepper, to taste
jacket potatoes, to serve
   (optional)

Heat a large frying pan (skillet) over a medium heat, add the curry paste and fry for 1 minute before adding the chickpeas (garbanzo beans). Stir until the chickpeas are well coated in the paste, then remove from the heat and transfer to a large mixing bowl.

In a small bowl, mix together the mayonnaise, yoghurt and mango chutney.

Stir the yoghurt mixture into the curried chickpeas, along with the celery, apricots and almonds, then gently stir in the coriander (cilantro). Season to taste.

Serve with salad leaves, as a wrap/sandwich filling, as a topping for jacket potatoes or as a side dish at a barbecue.

Salmon and Sweet Potato Fishcakes

Fishcakes are one of my favourite meals; however, I hate it when they are covered in breadcrumbs and contain very little fish, like many store-bought versions. Using sweet potato slightly increases the carb count in these homemade fishcakes, but they also work with white potatoes (or a mixture) and are nice served with peas. The orange colour of sweet potatoes comes from beta carotene, a powerful antioxidant that helps protect cells from sun damage – perfect if you have a long run outside – though don't skip the suncream!

SERVES 4

2 x 150-g (5½-oz) salmon fillets
500g (1lb 2oz) sweet potatoes, peeled and roughly chopped
large handful fresh coriander (cilantro), roughly chopped
4 spring onions (scallions)
1 red chilli, finely chopped (optional)
3 lemons: 1 zested; 1 juiced and zested; 1 cut into wedges to serve
1 Tbsp olive oil
150g (5½oz/¾ cup) full-fat Greek yoghurt
salt and freshly ground black pepper, to taste

Preheat the oven to 180°C/350°F/gas mark 4.

Put the salmon fillets on a baking sheet and bake for 10–12 minutes, or until cooked through. Remove from the oven and set aside.

Meanwhile, bring a large saucepan of water to the boil, add the sweet potatoes and cook for 15 minutes or until soft. Drain the potatoes into a sieve or colander.

Transfer the drained potatoes to a food processor and blitz briefly, before adding the coriander (cilantro), most of the spring onions (scallions), all the chilli and the zest from 1 of the lemons. Pulse to mix. Flake in the salmon and pulse briefly, being careful not to overmix. Season to taste and shape into 8 patties. Chill in the refrigerator for 30 minutes, if you have time.

When ready to cook, heat the oil in a large frying pan (skillet) over a medium heat, add the patties and fry for 5 minutes on each side until golden. You may need to do this in batches, keeping the cooked fishcakes warm while you cook the rest.

In a small bowl, mix the yoghurt with the juice and zest from 1 of the lemons and the remaining spring onions. Add plenty of seasoning.

Serve the fishcakes alongside the yoghurt dip, with lemon wedges to garnish and seasonal vegetables, if you like.

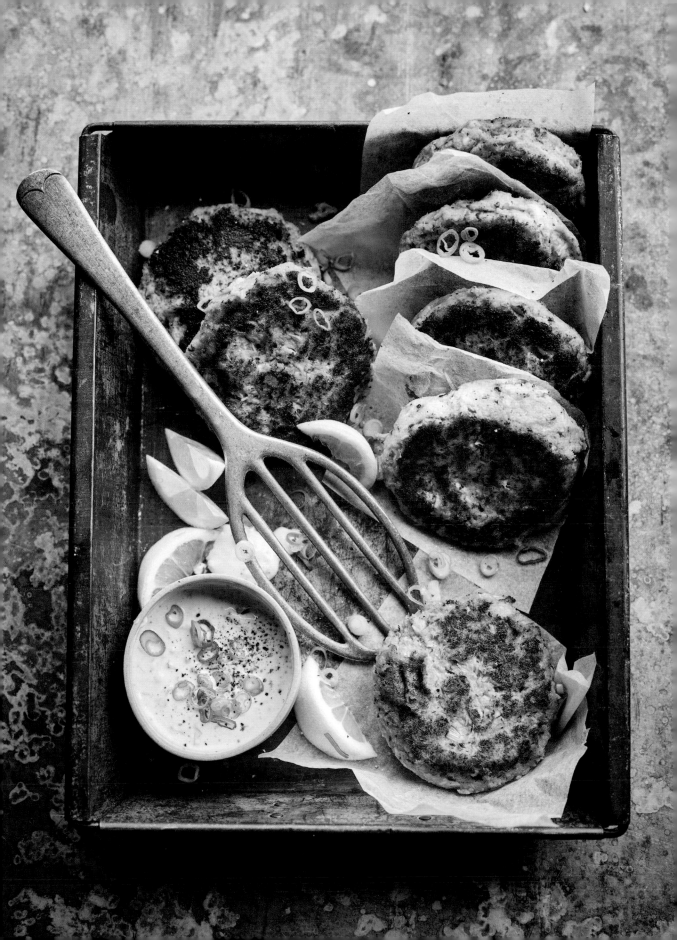

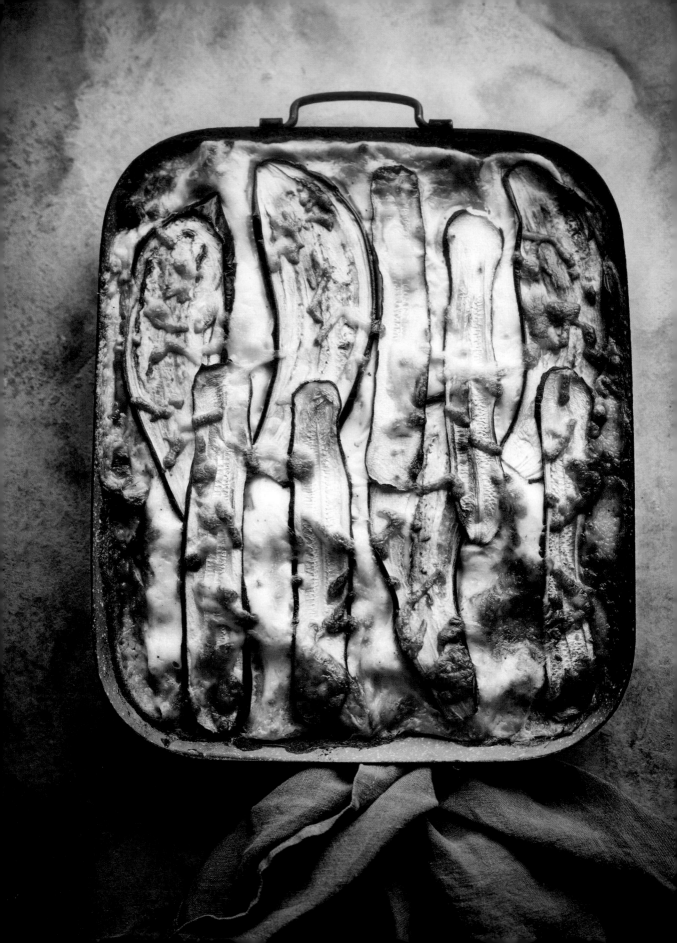

Veggie-Filled Lasagne

This doesn't lose any of the comfort of a traditional lasagne, but there's a whole load of veggies smuggled in too. If you're trying to cut down on your red meat consumption, you could use minced (ground) turkey or Quorn mince instead. Personally, if I'm using Quorn, I'll often add a drop or two (actually about 200ml/7fl oz/scant 1 cup) of red wine for added flavour, allowing the alcohol to burn off over a high heat for a couple of minutes.

SERVES 6

2 courgettes (zucchini), thinly sliced lengthways
1 large aubergine (eggplant), thinly sliced lengthways
1 tsp olive oil
1 onion, finely chopped
2 cloves garlic, finely chopped
400g (14oz) extra-lean minced (ground) beef
200g (7oz) mushrooms, roughly chopped
2 large carrots, coarsely grated
1 x 400-g (14-oz) can chopped tomatoes
1 Tbsp tomato purée (paste)
1 Tbsp dried mixed herbs
few dashes Worcestershire sauce
80g (3oz/⅓ cup) butter
40g (1½oz/generous ¼ cup) plain (all-purpose) flour
850ml (29fl oz/3½ cups) milk
6 dried lasagne sheets
50g (2oz/½ cup) Cheddar cheese, coarsely grated
salt and freshly ground black pepper, to taste
crisp green salad, to serve

Preheat the grill (broiler) to high.

Lay the courgette (zucchini) and aubergine (eggplant) slices in a single layer on baking sheets. Season with salt and grill (broil) for 2–3 minutes on each side until cooked through. Set aside on paper towels to remove any excess moisture.

Meanwhile, heat the oil in a large saucepan over a low heat, add the onion and cook for about 10 minutes until soft. Increase the heat, add the garlic and beef and cook for 5 minutes, stirring frequently, then add the mushrooms and carrots and cook for a further 5 minutes. Add the tomatoes, tomato purée (paste), herbs and Worcestershire sauce, season to taste and bring to the boil, then reduce the heat and simmer for 15 minutes, stirring occasionally. Check the seasoning, remove from the heat and set aside.

Preheat the oven to 200°C/400°F/gas mark 6.

In a separate saucepan, melt the butter, then stir in the flour and cook for 1 minute. Remove from the heat, then gradually stir in the milk until well combined and lump-free. Return to the heat and, stirring frequently, bring to the boil. Let bubble and thicken for a few minutes, then remove from the heat and season to taste.

Spoon half of the meat sauce into a large ovenproof baking dish, about 20 x 40cm (8 x 16in), top with half of the grilled vegetables, in an even layer, then top with a layer of the dried pasta sheets. Spoon over half of the white sauce, then repeat the layering with the remaining meat sauce, veg, pasta and white sauce. Top with the grated cheese.

Bake for 30–35 minutes or until piping hot and golden on top. Serve immediately with a crisp green salad.

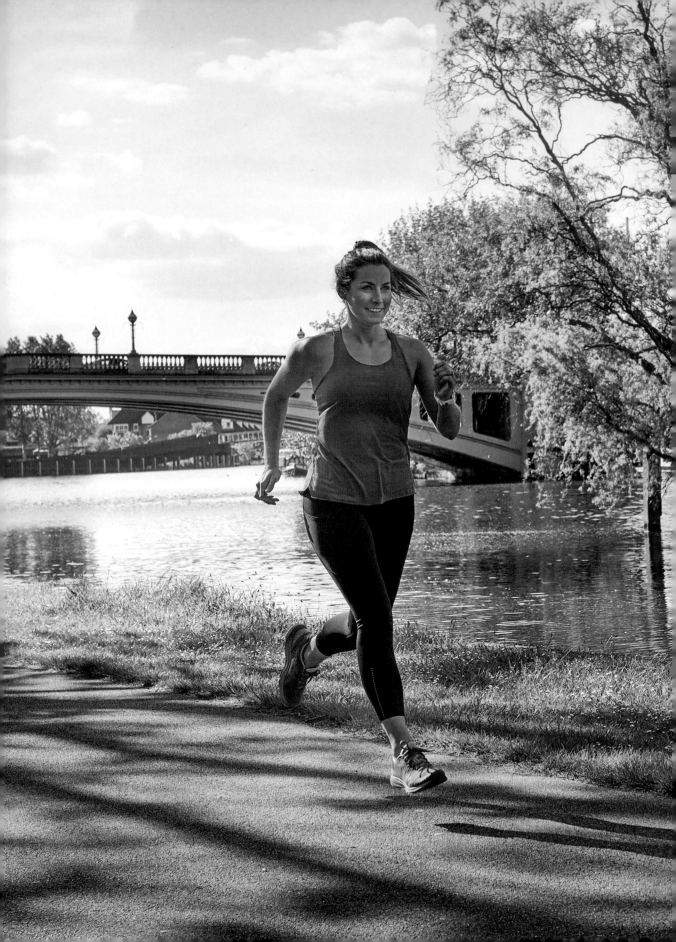

REFUEL – SWEET

It's no secret that a lot of runners say they 'run to eat', or in particular that they 'run for cake'. I often meet a friend for a run and follow it up with coffee and cake. I've created some recipes that will hit that sweet treat craving, but will also help you refuel after your workout. They include protein, carbs and fat, as well as some extra nutrients from the fruit and veg I've sneaked into some of the bakes!

After a long run or hard workout, it's important to try to consume 20–30g (⅔–1oz) protein to help you repair and build muscle. It was previoulsy thought that we had to consume this protein within 30 minutes of finishing our workout, although new research suggests that it doesn't matter when exactly you consume your protein as long as you meet your daily requirement. This can be done through snacks, meals and drinks.

However, you don't just need protein – it's key to replenish glycogen stores with carbohydrates. This is best done with a combination of protein and carbs for glycogen synthesesis. You are looking for a ratio of 3:1 of carbs to protein, and they don't have to come from a protein bar or shake.

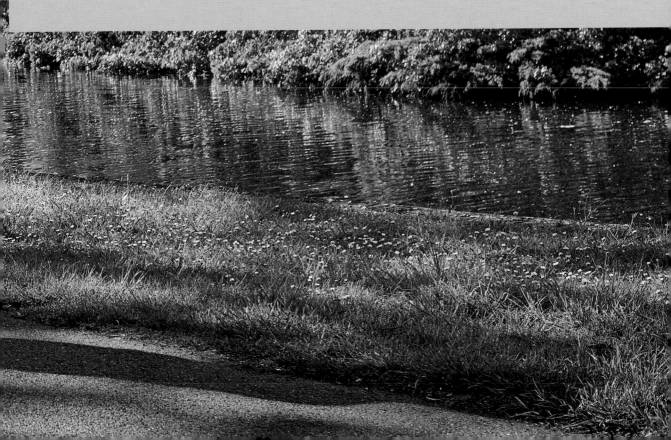

Iced Latte Cubes

Semi-skimmed milk does a great job as a post-run refuel drink. In the summer, I find nothing more refreshing than getting an iced latte on the way back from my run – the coffee shop baristas are used to my sweaty post-run look at 7a.m.! This post-run refresher packs in over 17g ($\frac{2}{3}$oz) carbs and 12g ($\frac{1}{2}$oz) protein when served with cow's milk. It's perfect served with one of the breakfast recipes or a Monster Workout Cookie (see page 123)!

Silicone ice trays tend to work best for making these coffee cubes, to keep them intact, but you can pick whatever shape you like!

MAKES ENOUGH FOR 3–4 LATTES

2 shots espresso
    (or 2 coffee pods)

To serve (per drink):
350ml (12fl oz/1½ cups)
    semi-skimmed milk, or a
    dairy-free milk, if preferred

First make your coffee, pour it into an ice cube tray and freeze until solid. I tend to make a large batch of these at a time. If you prefer a weaker latte, dilute your espresso down before freezing.

To serve, add 2–3 coffee cubes to a glass of milk and let them melt. If you like a stronger latte, simply add more ice cubes to your glass of milk.

If you prefer your coffee blended, blitz together the milk and ice cubes in a blender until you reach the desired consistency.

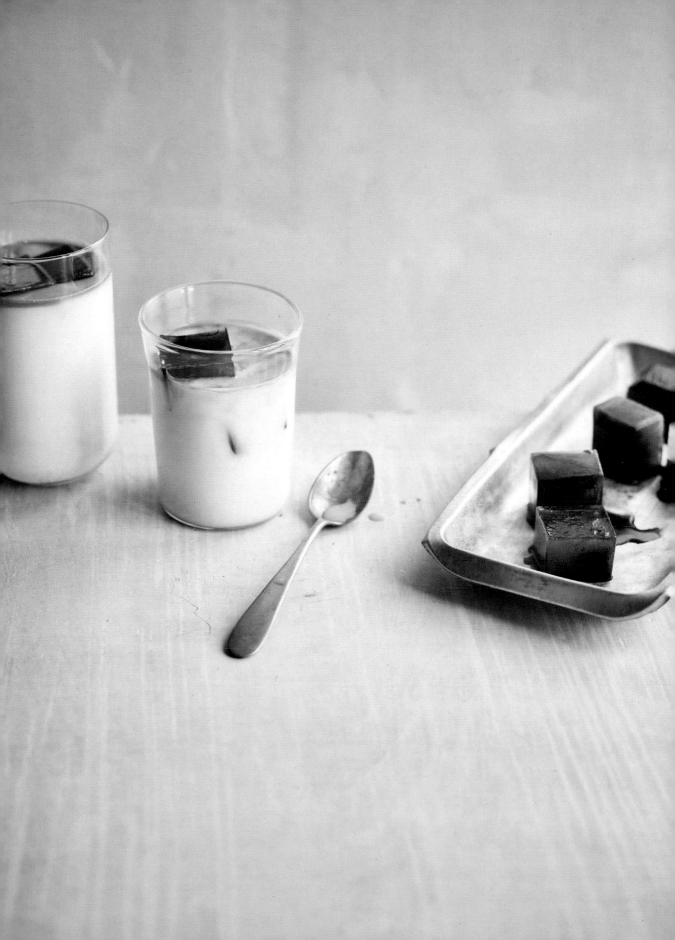

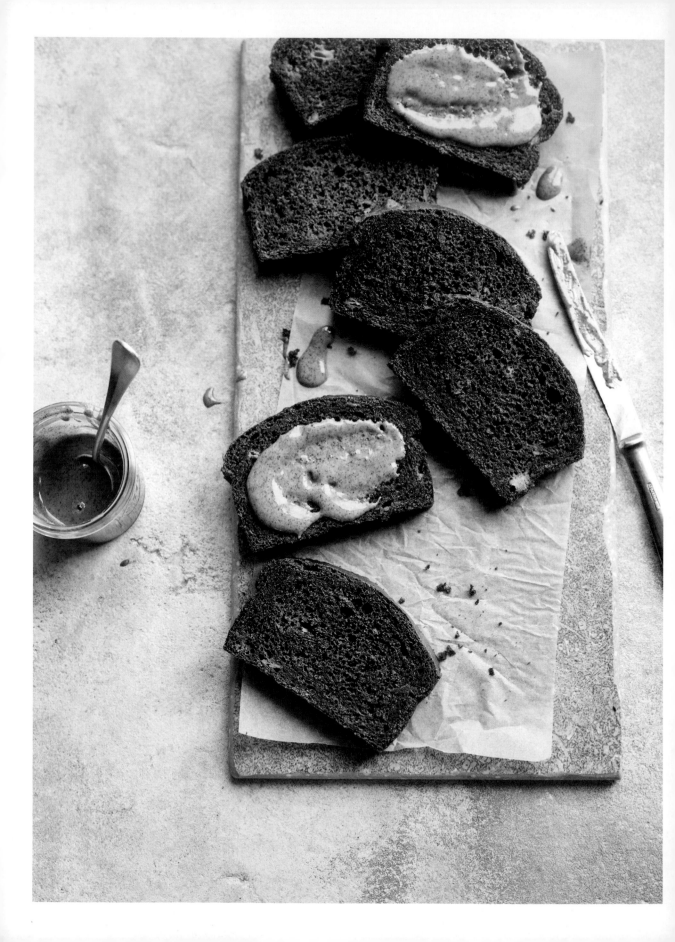

Triple Chocolate Banana Bread

Does anyone else purposefully buy extra bananas, just so they can let them go brown and then they will *have* to make banana bread? Well, if not, I hope this recipe will make you start! This is delicious served solo or with a generous dollop of nut butter (especially when the loaf is a few days old). My friends ate the testing batches for breakfast while on holiday in New Zealand and can confirm that it goes down pretty well at any time of day.

SERVES 8–10

125g (4½oz/scant 1 cup) plain (all-purpose) flour
50g (2oz/6 Tbsp) oat flour (or blitz jumbo/old-fashioned oats in a food processor until fine)
2 Tbsp cocoa powder
1 tsp baking powder
1 tsp bicarbonate of soda (baking soda)
2 large ripe bananas
75g (2⅔oz/6 Tbsp) soft brown sugar
1 medium egg
1 tsp vanilla extract
150g (5½oz/¾ cup) full-fat Greek yoghurt
100g (3½oz/7 Tbsp) unsalted butter, melted
30g (1oz/3 Tbsp) white chocolate chips
30g (1oz/3 Tbsp) milk chocolate chips

Preheat the oven to 180°C/350°F/gas mark 4 and line a 900-g (2-lb) loaf tin (pan) with baking paper.

In a large bowl, mix together the flours, cocoa powder, baking powder and bicarbonate of soda (baking soda).

In a separate bowl, thoroughly mash the bananas. Stir in the sugar, egg, vanilla and yoghurt, then carefully stir in the melted butter (make sure it's not too hot so the egg doesn't cook).

Mix the wet ingredients into the dry until just combined, then stir in the chocolate chips.

Pour the batter into the prepared tin and bake for 55–60 minutes, or until an inserted skewer comes out clean.

Leave to cool in the tin for 20 minutes before turning out onto a wire rack to cool completely. Alternatively, you can cut it carefully and serve slightly gooey. It's perfect after a long run, with a cuppa!

Avocado Loaf

This loaf gives the avocado-on-toast obsession new meaning, although I have to admit that I haven't tried this with a poached egg and chilli flakes on top!

SERVES 8–10

75g (2⅔oz/⅓ cup) unsalted butter, softened

175g (6oz/¾ cup) golden caster (superfine) sugar

150g (5½oz) very ripe avocado, mashed

juice and finely grated zest of 1 lemon

2 medium eggs, whisked

200g (7oz/1½ cups) wholemeal flour

pinch salt

1 tsp baking powder

1 tsp bicarbonate of soda (baking soda)

100g (3½oz/½ cup) full-fat Greek yoghurt

Preheat the oven to 180°C/350°F/gas mark 4 and line a 900-g (2-lb) loaf tin (pan) with baking paper.

In a large bowl, use an electric hand-mixer to whisk together the butter and sugar until light and fluffy. Mix in the mashed avocado and lemon juice and zest. Slowly, a little at a time, add the beaten eggs to the mix, whisking to combine.

In a separate large bowl, sift together the flour, salt, baking powder and bicarbonate of soda (baking soda).

Fold half of the flour mixture into the wet ingredients before folding in the yoghurt, followed by the remaining flour mixture.

Spoon the batter into the prepared tin and bake for 55–60 minutes, or until an inserted skewer comes out clean.

Leave to cool in the tin for a few minutes before turning out onto a wire rack to cool completely. Cut into slices and serve.

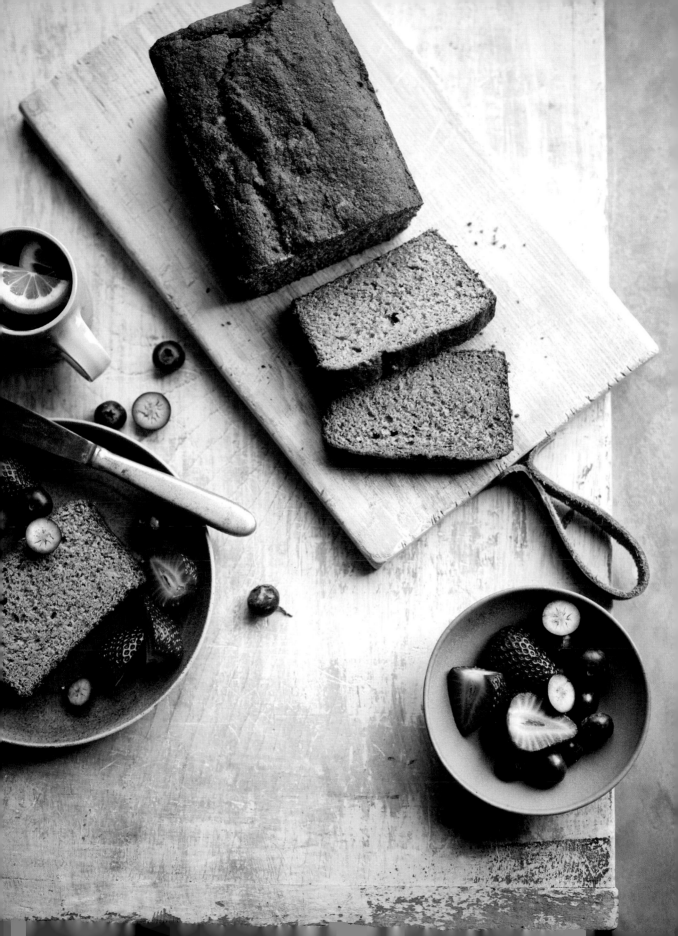

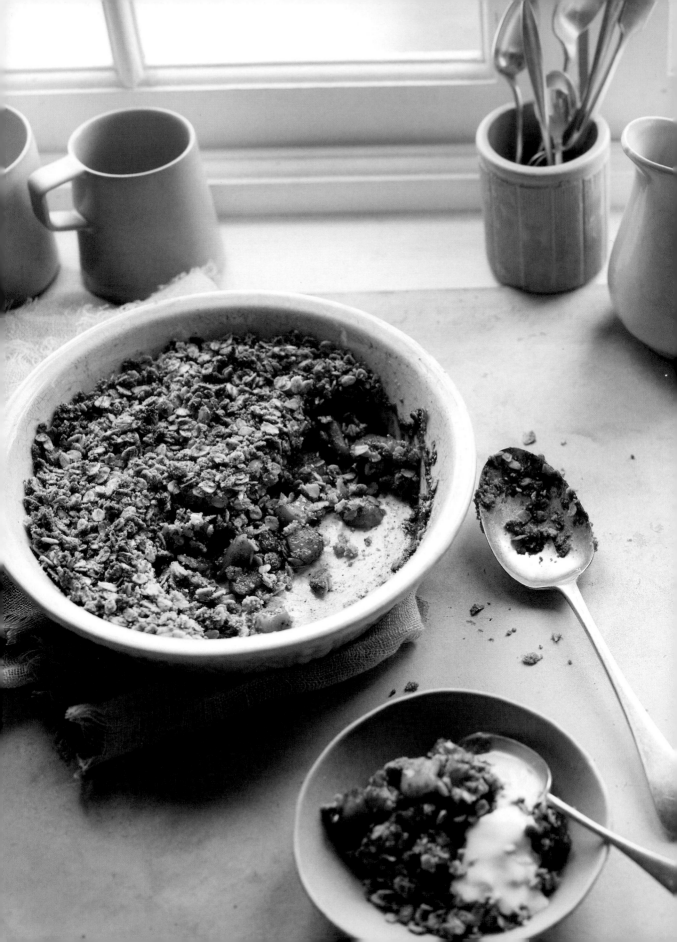

Pear and Apple Crumble

Crumble has a special place in my heart. To be honest, I almost put this in the breakfast section of the book because that's my favourite time of the day to eat crumble! Maybe that's why I was so keen to put oats in the topping. This is great at any time of the day, served with a big dollop of creamy Greek yoghurt or frozen yoghurt, or – if you ask my husband Tom – with double (heavy) cream or ice cream. You choose.

SERVES 6–8

3 pears (I like Packham's pears), peeled and roughly chopped

3 eating apples, peeled and roughly chopped

50g (2oz/¼ cup) light brown muscovado sugar

1 tsp ground cardamon or ground ginger

2 tsp ground cinnamon

50ml (1⅔fl oz/3½ Tbsp) melted coconut oil

50g (2oz/½ cup) ground almonds

100g (3½oz/1 cup) rolled (old-fashioned) porridge oats

Greek yoghurt or dairy-free alternative, to serve (optional)

In a large saucepan, mix together the pears and apples with 1 tablespoon of the sugar, the ground cardamon or ginger, and 1 teaspoon of the cinnamon. Cook over a low heat for 15 minutes until the sugar melts and the fruit is just beginning to soften.

Meanwhile, make the crumble topping. In a large bowl, mix together the melted coconut oil with the remaining sugar and cinnamon, and the ground almonds and oats.

Spoon the cooked fruit mixture into a deep baking dish (about 22-cm (8½-in) square or thereabouts), and cover with the oat crumble topping. Bake for 40–45 minutes or until the top is crispy and golden. Serve immediately with Greek yoghurt, or your preferred accompaniment.

Super Runner Loaf

I was hugely inspired by running superstar Shalane Flanagan's book *Run Fast, Cook Fast, Eat Slow* (co-written with Elyse Kopecky). This recipe is a tribute to their Superhero Muffins – I've shaped it into an easy-slice loaf and added chocolate chips because, duh, chocolate is amazing. For those who aren't fans of Shalane Flanagan, she won the New York City Marathon in 2017 (the first American to win since 1977), and came third on the same course in 2018. She is a four-time Olympian, earning an Olympic Silver Medal in the 10K in 2008. But my favourite thing about her is her relationship with and unwavering support of other athletes, in particular female runners. She's paced a number of her fellow Nike Bowerman Track Club runners to big PBs (and even an American record!) on the track.

SERVES 8–10

200g (7oz/2 cups) ground almonds
125g (4½oz/1¼ cups) quick-cook porridge oats (instant oatmeal)
50g (2oz/generous ⅓ cup) raisins
50g (2oz/½ cup) chopped pecans
2 tsp ground cinnamon
½ tsp ground nutmeg
1 tsp bicarbonate of soda (baking soda)
pinch salt
3 medium eggs, lightly beaten
1 large courgette (zucchini), coarsely grated
1 large carrot, coarsely grated
75g (2⅔oz/⅓ cup) unsalted butter, melted
50ml (1⅔fl oz/3½ Tbsp) maple syrup
1 tsp vanilla extract
50g (2oz/⅓ cup) chocolate chips

Preheat the oven to 200°C/400°F/gas mark 6 and line a 900-g (2-lb) loaf tin (pan) with baking paper.

In a large bowl, mix together the ground almonds, oats, raisins, pecans, cinnamon, nutmeg, bicarbonate of soda (baking soda) and salt.

In a separate bowl, mix together the eggs, courgette (zucchini), carrot, melted butter, maple syrup and vanilla extract.

Stir the wet ingredients into the dry ingredients, then add in the chocolate chips, mixing until just combined.

Pour the batter into the prepared tin and bake for 55–60 minutes, or until an inserted skewer comes out clean.

Leave to cool in the tin for 10 minutes before carefully turning out onto a wire rack to cool completely.

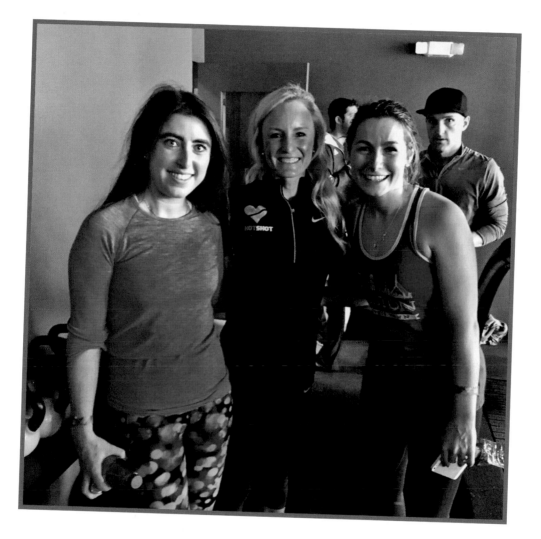

Photo taken at Heartbreak Hill Running Company of Zoe Meskell (left),
Shalane Flanagan (middle) and myself, Boston 2017.

Choc-o'Clock Sweet Potato Brownies

The healthy-eating blogger Deliciously Ella made adding veg to your brownies cool back in 2015, when her sweet potato brownie recipe was a huge hit. However, I don't make these healthy brownies to cut down on the sugar and butter (because there is definitely a time and a place for a 'proper' brownie); instead, I love them because they are packed full of slow-release energy to help you go from your 4p.m. cup of tea and choccie in the office to your evening gym session or run without getting that post-treat energy slump.

I roast up a couple of sweet potatoes most Sunday evenings as they keep in the fridge for up to a week and make for super-quick, easy lunches; they can be added to recipes such as fishcakes, or used for baking.

MAKES 9

400g (14oz) cooked sweet potato

140g (5oz/½ cup) agave nectar

100g (3½oz/scant ½ cup) almond butter

120ml (4fl oz/½ cup) coconut oil, melted

2 tsp vanilla extract or scraped seeds from 1 vanilla pod

80g (3oz/¾ cup) cacao powder or cocoa powder

70g (2½oz/½ cup) plain (all-purpose) flour

80g (3oz/½ cup) chocolate chips, or dairy-free alternative

Preheat the oven to 200°C/400°F/gas mark 6 and line a 23-cm (9-in) square cake tin (brownie pan) with baking paper.

In a large bowl, thoroughly mash the sweet potato, then stir in the agave nectar, almond butter, coconut oil and vanilla. Sift in the cacao or cocoa powder and flour and fold in, then stir in the chocolate chips.

Pour the batter into the prepared tin and level – the mixture is quite thick and needs to be spread evenly. Bake for 20 minutes, or until the crust is solid and browning on the top.

Leave to cool in the tin for 10 minutes before turning out onto a wire rack to cool completely. Cut into 9 squares and serve, either with a cup of tea or with berries and ice cream for a delicious dessert.

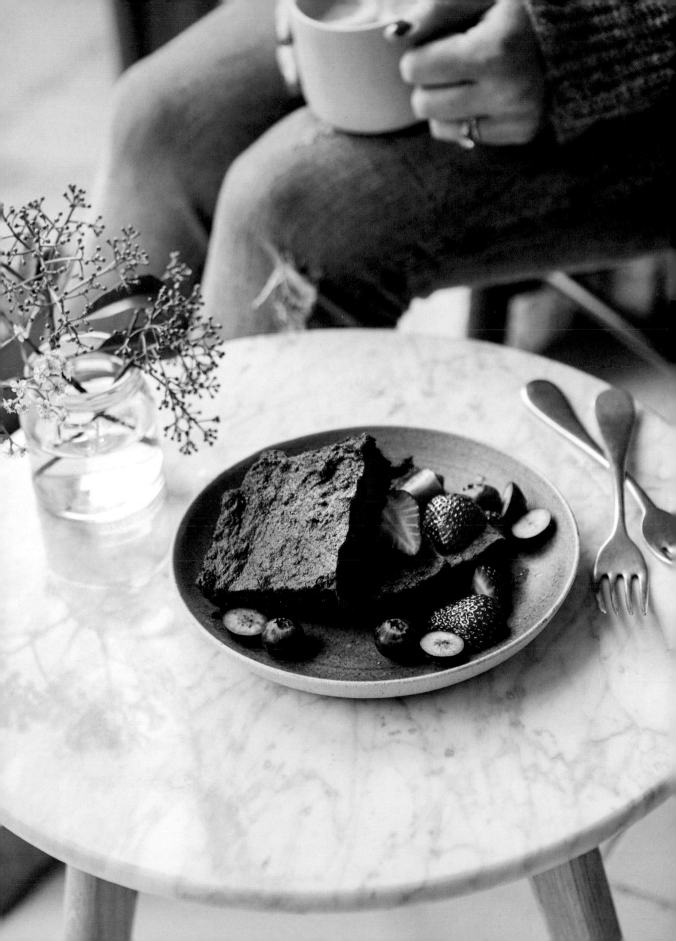

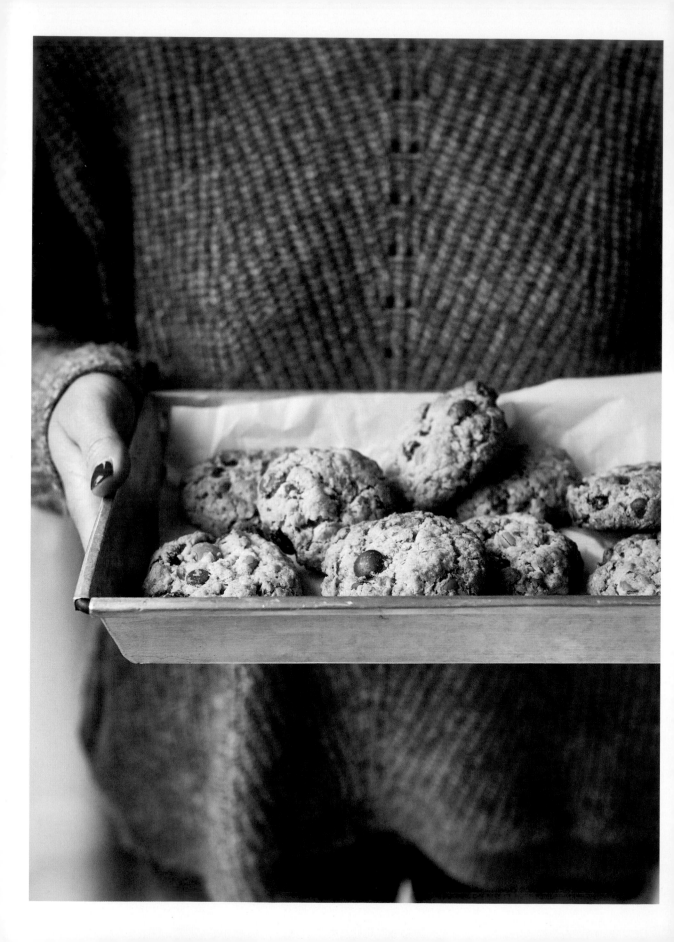

Monster Workout Cookies

Full disclosure – these are full-sugar cookies. I tried to reduce the sugar, but decided after some very rigorous testing, and 'constructive criticism' from my uncle James, that they just didn't cut it. So, yes, these are proper cookies, but the oats and peanut butter should at least tide you over a little longer than a regular cookie. Anyway, sometimes only the real deal will do.

Best enjoyed in an Epsom-salt bath with a cup of tea, speaking from experience.

MAKES 18

125g (4½oz/generous ½ cup) unsalted butter, softened
150g (5½oz/¾ cup) light brown soft sugar
50g (2oz/¼ cup) caster (superfine) sugar
100g (3½oz/½ cup) unsweetened, chunky peanut butter
1 large egg, lightly beaten
1 tsp vanilla extract
150g (5½oz/1 cup plus 2 Tbsp) plain (all-purpose) flour
125g (4½oz/1¼ cups) quick-cook porridge oats (instant oatmeal)
½ tsp baking powder
pinch salt
80g (3oz/⅓ cup) M&M's or Smarties sweets (chocolate candies)
50g (2oz/⅓ cup) chocolate chips
50g (2oz/generous ⅓ cup) sultanas (golden raisins)

Preheat the oven to 180°C/350°F/gas mark 4 and line 2 baking sheets with baking paper.

In a large bowl, use an electric handmixer to beat together the butter and sugars for 5 minutes until light and creamy, then beat in the peanut butter, egg and vanilla extract until well combined.

In a separate bowl, mix together the flour, oats, baking powder and salt. Carefully stir the dry ingredients into the wet until just combined, trying not to overmix. Finally, stir in the sweets (candies), chocolate chips and sultanas (golden raisins).

Dollop 9 spoonfuls of batter onto each prepared baking sheet (about 1 tablespoon per cookie), pressing down to spread the mixture slightly and leaving a gap between each cookie. Bake for 12–15 minutes until golden.

Leave to cool on the baking sheet for 10 minutes before transferring to a wire rack to cool completely.

Coconut Refresher Lollies

Forget the post-run electrolyte drink: swap it for a delicious and refreshing fruity ice lolly instead.

MAKES 6

100g (3½oz) mixed fresh or frozen fruit (I use blueberries, strawberries, mango and kiwi), chopped into very small, bite-size pieces
300ml (10fl oz/1¼ cups) coconut water

Make sure your fruit is chopped small enough to easily fit into your ice lolly moulds. Distribute the fruit evenly between 6 moulds, filling them to the top without overflowing. Carefully pour the coconut water over the fruit and cover with the lids (adding lolly sticks, if needed).

Freeze overnight, or for at least 8 hours.

To remove the lollies from the moulds, run them under warm running water for a few seconds and they should easily release. Enjoy immediately. Foam rolling while eating them is optional!

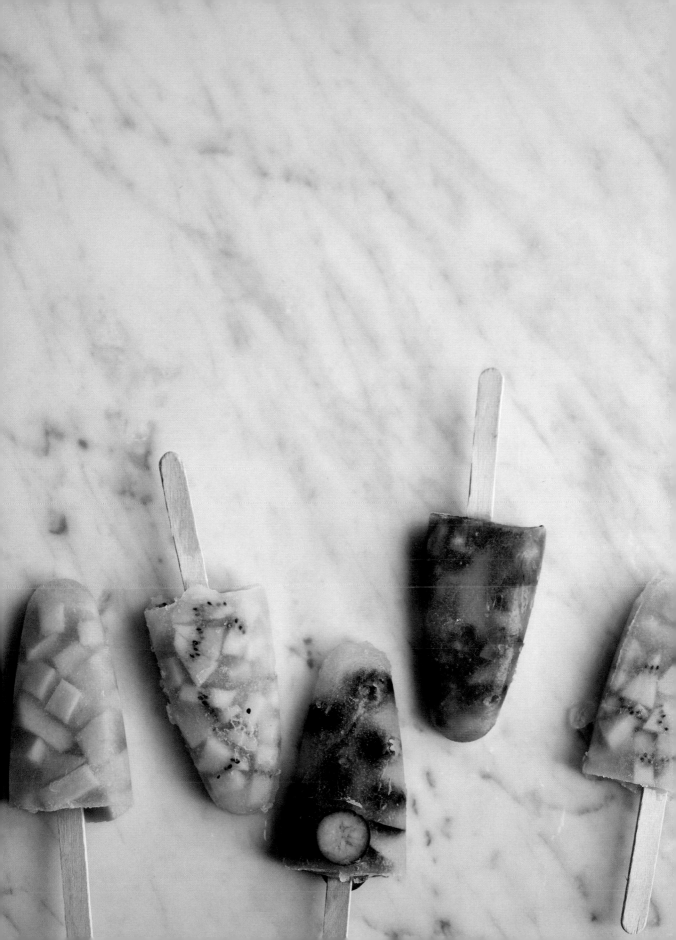

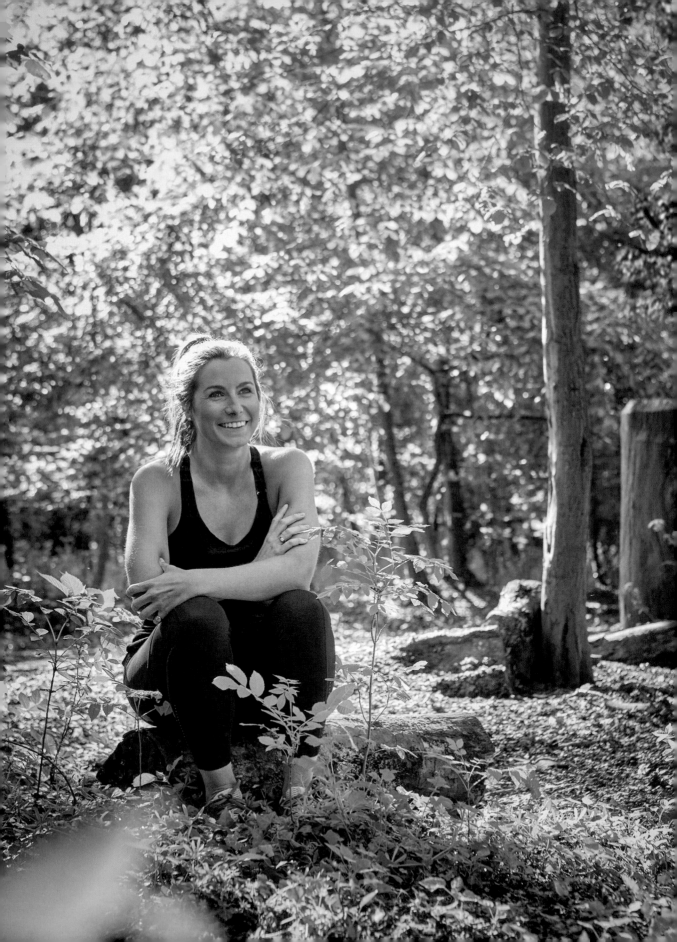

REFUEL – SAVOURY

Recovery.

I was once told that you should only run the number of miles that you can recover from. That means sleeping, stretching and, crucially, rehydrating and refuelling.

Rehydrating can be with a combination of water and/or electrolyte drinks, such as the ones found on page 45. You'll want around 500ml (17fl oz/generous 2 cups) post-race, then drink little and often throughout the rest of the day – more if you've sweated a lot or it's a hot day. You can test your approximate sweat rate by following the instructions on page 22.

Refuel with a combination of protein and carbohydrates. Protein is involved with muscle repair and adaptation (increased strength and power), making sure hard sessions actually make a difference in training. Athletes have higher daily protein needs than non-athletes, with requirements between 1.2–2g protein per kg of bodyweight per day (according to the American College of Sports Medicine). You should aim to get around 20g (¾oz) protein post-session, then eat regular protein as part of snacks and meals throughout the remainder of the day.

We also need carbohydrates to replace muscle glycogen, especially on longer runs. Studies have shown that if you have 24 hours of recovery between sessions, then eating your carbohydrates as meals and snacks according to your own schedule and preference is more than adequate. This can be in various forms – a combination of simple and complex carbohydrates found in sourdough or whole wheat bread, pasta, grains, beans, fruits, vegetables, etc.

However, if you have less than 8 hours between sessions (when doing two-a-day runs or workouts) or if you're doing one late-night session followed by an early morning workout, then you should try to consume adequate carbohydrates as soon as possible after your first workout. Opt for carbohydrate-rich foods with a mid–high glycemic index for muscle glycogen synthesis. These are carbohydrates that break down quickly, such as potatoes, rice, white bread, honey and starchy vegetables – just like the recipes you'll find in this chapter.

Post-Run Pie

This takes a while to make, but can be left to bubble on the stove or in a slow cooker while you go for a run (with someone else at home to check on it). Alternatively, make it in advance and refrigerate, then just bake when you're ready to go.

SERVES 6–8

750g (1lb 10oz) beef stewing steak, cut into 2.5-cm (1-in) cubes

3 Tbsp plain (all-purpose) flour

2 Tbsp olive oil, plus extra as needed

4 shallots, peeled and quartered

200g (7oz) button mushrooms, halved if large

4 sprigs fresh thyme

2 carrots, roughly chopped

400ml (14fl oz/1⅔ cups) beef stock (bouillon)

200ml (7fl oz/scant 1 cup) red wine (optional, swap for beef stock/bouillon if you prefer)

1kg (2lb 3oz) potatoes, peeled and roughly chopped

3 parsnips, peeled and roughly chopped

1 Tbsp butter

40g (1½oz/½ cup) Cheddar cheese, coarsely grated

salt and freshly ground black pepper, to taste

peas and seasonal veg, to serve

In a large bowl, toss the beef in the flour with plenty of seasoning. Heat half of the oil in a large heavy saucepan (with a lid) over a medium-high heat and brown half of the beef. Remove using a slotted spoon and set aside. Repeat with the remaining oil and beef, then remove and set aside.

In the same pan, fry the shallots and mushrooms for 10 minutes until softened (add a little extra oil if the pan looks too dry). Return the beef to the pan, then add the thyme, carrots, stock (bouillon) and wine, if using. Bring to the boil, then reduce the heat to low, cover and simmer gently for 1¼–1½ hours, until the beef is tender.

Preheat the oven to 200°C/400°F/gas mark 6.

Meanwhile, put the potatoes and parsnips in a large saucepan and cover with cold water. Bring to the boil, then reduce to a simmer and cook for 20 minutes or until completely soft. Drain, then add the butter to the veg in the pan and mash together until smooth.

Transfer the beef mixture to a deep baking or pie dish (about 30 x 23 x 6cm/12 x 9 x 2½in), top with the mash and sprinkle over the grated cheese. Bake for 20–25 minutes, or until the mixture is bubbling and the cheese is melted and golden.

Serve immediately with peas and seasonal veg.

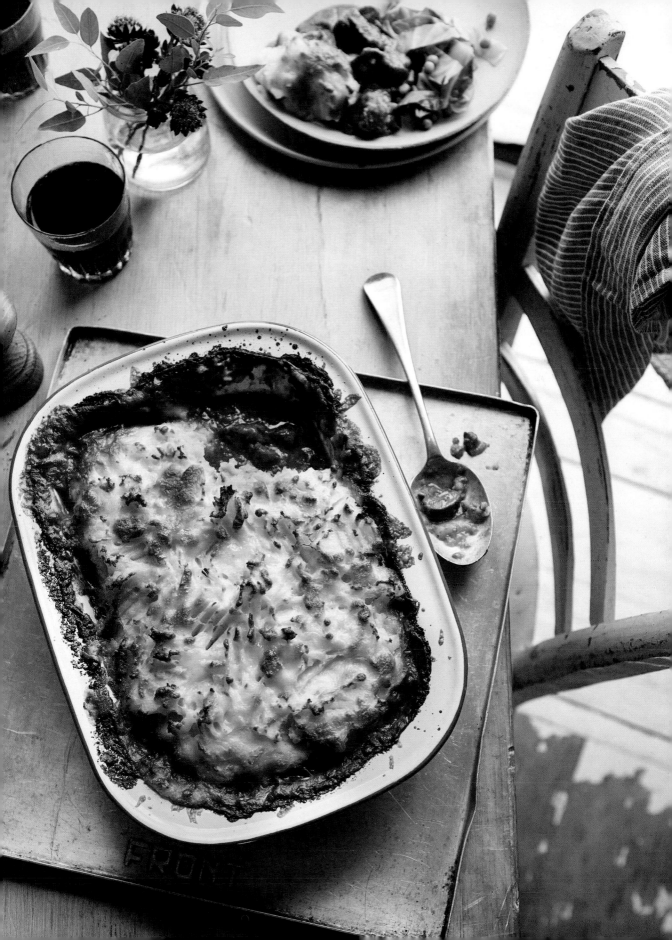

Chorizo Chilli

My friend Amanda made this for a girls' night dinner years ago, just after we had left uni and were trying to save money by eating out less. We would take it in turns to host, bringing multiple offerings of chips and dips and bottles of wine, and this chorizo chilli became a firm favourite. Amanda said her original recipe was 'a bit of this and a bit of that', so feel free to vary it depending on what's in your refrigerator, in season or on personal preference. It actually adds to the beauty of this dish – the butternut squash can easily be subbed for sweet potatoes, the quinoa swapped for pearl barley, and the (bell) pepper swapped out for courgette (zucchini). If you're anything like me and my friends, serve with a big bowl of guacamole, chips and even margaritas!

SERVES 4

75g (2⅔oz) chorizo, cut into small cubes
1 onion, finely sliced
1 red (bell) pepper, deseeded and roughly chopped
400g (14oz) butternut squash, chopped into 2.5-cm (1-in) cubes
2 cloves garlic, crushed
1 tsp paprika
1 tsp ground cumin
1 Tbsp tomato purée (paste)
200g (7oz/scant 1¼ cups) quinoa
1 x 400-g (14-oz) can chopped tomatoes
500ml (17fl oz/generous 2 cups) vegetable or chicken stock (bouillon)
1 x 400-g (14-oz) can kidney beans, drained

To serve:
1 avocado, sliced
handful fresh coriander (cilantro), chopped
about 4 Tbsp full-fat Greek yoghurt

Heat a large heavy pan over a high heat, add the chorizo and fry for 5 minutes, turning occasionally, until golden and its oil has been released. Using a slotted spoon, remove the chorizo and set aside, leaving the oil behind in the pan.

Add the onion, (bell) pepper and butternut squash to the chorizo oil and fry for 8 minutes or until soft, then add the garlic, spices and tomato purée (paste) and fry for a further minute. Stir in the quinoa and fry for another minute, then add the chopped tomatoes and stock (bouillon) and bring to the boil. Reduce the heat to a simmer and let bubble for 15 minutes, or until the quinoa is cooked and the mixture has thickened. Add a little water if it's getting too thick.

Stir the chorizo back in, along with the kidney beans, and heat through.

Serve with sliced avocado, fresh coriander (cilantro) and a dollop of Greek yoghurt and season to taste.

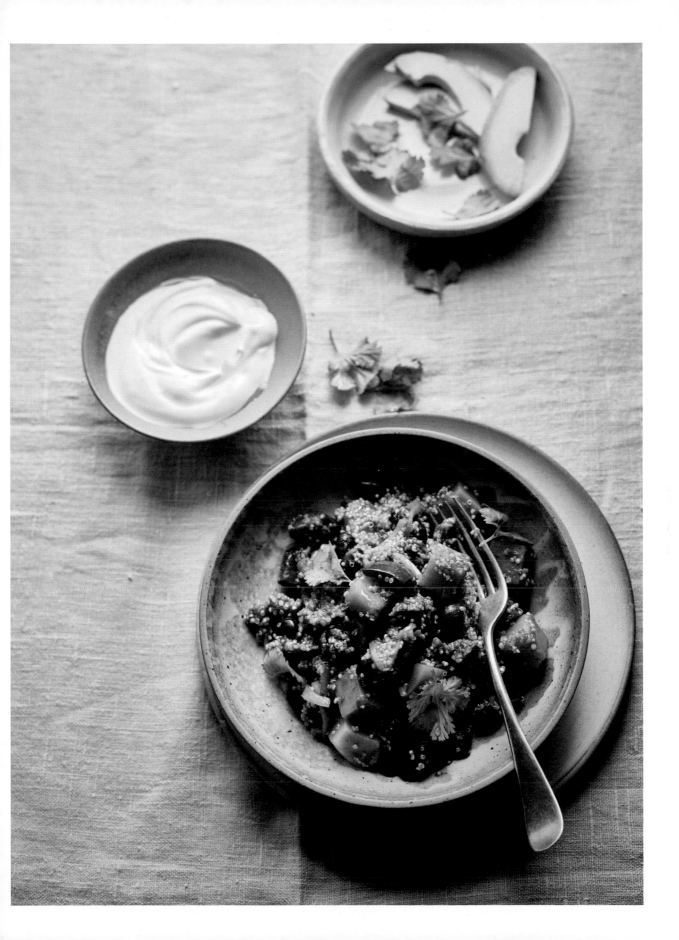

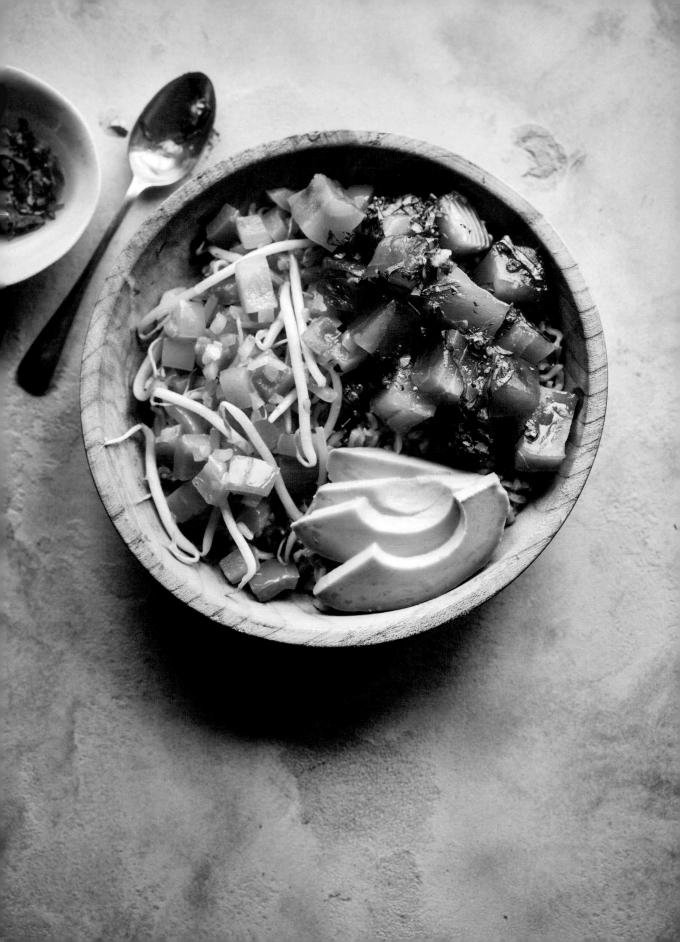

EAT LIKE AN ELITE

Kara Goucher's Poke Bowl

Kara Goucher recently claimed her silver medal from the IAAF World Championships, having been awarded the bronze medal in Osaka in 2007. She ran her first 26.2 at the New York City Marathon in 2008, placing third and running what was, at the time, the fastest-ever American women's marathon debut. In her Chicago Half Marathon win in 2009 she came from 30th place in the final mile, and won in 1.08.05 – the fastest anyone ran that day, male or female.

SERVES 4 (OR 2 HUNGRY RUNNERS!)

250g (9oz/1¼ cups) brown rice
450g (1lb) sushi-grade tuna or salmon, diced into large chunks (leave in one piece if cooking)
1 Tbsp olive oil or avocado oil
1 onion, finely chopped
2 (bell) peppers (any colour), deseeded and roughly chopped
250g (9oz) bean sprouts
1 avocado, sliced, to serve

For the sauce:
1–2 cloves garlic, crushed
small handful fresh basil, finely chopped
juice of 1 lime
60ml (2fl oz/¼ cup) fish sauce
2 Tbsp sweet chilli sauce
50ml (2fl oz/¼ cup) olive oil or avocado oil
salt and freshly ground black pepper, to taste

Cook the rice according to the packet instructions.

Meanwhile, mix together the sauce ingredients in a small bowl, adding salt and pepper to taste, and set aside.

If you prefer to serve your fish raw (as poke is traditionally served), simply cube it and set aside.

If you prefer to cook your fish, preheat the oven to 200°C/400°F/gas mark 6.

Heat an ovenproof frying pan (skillet) over a medium-high heat with a little of the oil and sear the fish for 2 minutes on each side. Transfer to the oven to cook for 8–12 minutes, depending on how thick the fish is and how well you like it cooked. Once cooked, dice the fish.

Heat the remaining oil in a separate pan over a medium-high heat, add the onion and (bell) peppers and sauté until just tender. Stir through the bean sprouts and cook for a further 3–5 minutes. Season with salt and pepper to taste.

Once the rice is cooked, the veggies are sautéed and the fish is ready, you can build your poke bowl. Start with a serving of brown rice, then top with the veggies, add the fish and pour over a small amount of the sauce. Serve the rest of the sauce on the side – you can always add more to taste. Finally, top with some avocado slices and enjoy!

Pistachio-Crusted Salmon

This dish is ideal for when friends come over for a weekend supper. The pistachio crust also works well with flaky white fish, such as cod, and my non-fish-loving husband can also confirm that it works well spread on a chicken breast, too!

Long-stem broccoli or mangetout (snow peas) are also delicious in place of the pak choi (bok choy) – just cook until tender.

SERVES 4

4 x 125-g (4½-oz) salmon fillets or 1 large salmon piece (about 500g/1lb 2oz)
2 tsp runny honey
3 Tbsp soy sauce
2 aubergines (eggplants), sliced into rounds 2cm (¾in) thick, flesh scored in a criss-cross pattern
1½ tsp olive oil
1 large clove garlic, crushed
200g (7oz) pak choi (bok choy), trimmed, separated, washed and patted dry
1 spring onion (scallion), finely chopped
zest of 1 lemon
cooked brown rice and lemon wedges, to serve

For the pistachio crust:
1½ Tbsp olive oil
75g (2⅔oz/generous ½ cup) shelled pistachios
2 spring onions (scallions), finely chopped
2 tsp runny honey

Preheat the oven to 200°C/400°F/gas mark 6.

In a food processor, blitz together the pistachio crust ingredients to form a chunky paste.

Place the salmon fillet on a baking sheet. Spread the pistachio paste over the top of the salmon in a thick layer and set aside.

In a small bowl, mix together the honey with 2 tablespoons of the soy sauce. Place the aubergine (eggplant) slices on a large baking sheet and brush with half of the soy/honey mixture, then turn them over and brush the other sides. Drizzle any remaining soy/honey mixture over the top and roast for 25–30 minutes until softened.

Add the salmon to the oven for the final 12–15 minutes of cooking time, until it is just cooked and the pistachio crust is beginning to brown.

Meanwhile, heat the oil in a large frying pan (skillet) over a low-medium heat, add the garlic and fry for 1 minute. Add the pak choi (bok choy) and the remaining tablespoon of soy sauce and fry until softened, about 5 minutes. Remove from the heat and stir in the chopped spring onion (scallion) and lemon zest.

Serve the salmon, aubergine slices and pak choi with brown rice and lemon wedges on the side.

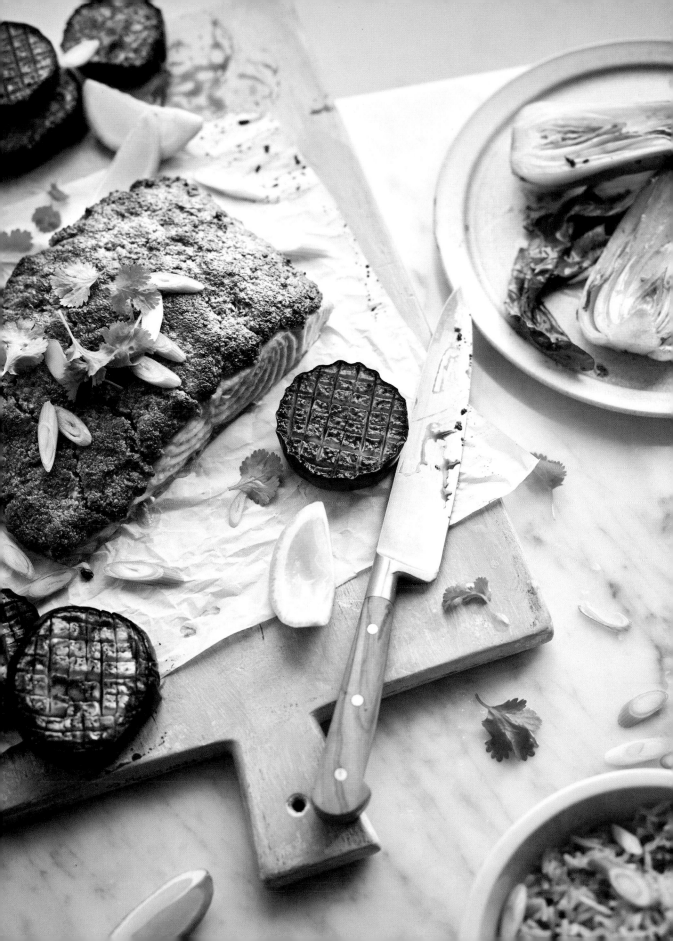

Miso Broccoli

Broccoli might be my favourite vegetable. This recipe came from my Aunt Sandra, who is an excellent cook; she can whip up something out of seemingly nothing. If you don't have miso paste, then a tablespoon of soy sauce is a good alternative. This also pairs well with the Pistachio-Crusted Salmon (pictured on page 135).

SERVES 4

1 medium head of broccoli or 300g (10½oz) long-stem broccoli
1½ tsp white miso paste
1 Tbsp sesame oil
2 Tbsp pine nuts
1 tsp black sesame seeds (optional)
juice of ½ lemon

Cut the broccoli into florets and don't waste the stem – just slice this after cutting off the tough bits. Bring a large pan of water to the boil and cook the broccoli for 3 minutes or until just softened. Alternatively, steam the broccoli until just cooked. Drain the broccoli and set aside briefly.

Gently warm the miso paste in the same saucepan, then add the cooked broccoli back to the pan along with the sesame oil. Toss until the broccoli is well coated and warmed through.

Check the seasoning, then transfer to a serving plate. Sprinkle over the pine nuts and sesame seeds (if using) and squeeze over the lemon juice. Serve immediately.

SUPERFOOD: SALMON

Salmon is not only a great protein source to fuel your body pre- and post-workout, but also one of the best food sources of omega-3 fats. Omega-3s are essential for brain development and function, and joint health, and also help prevent heart disease and high blood pressure. Athletes benefit from their anti-inflammatory properties, reducing inflammation at a cellular level to help reduce pain and soreness. Marine sources of omega-3s are most easily absorbed by the body.

Salmon is high in vitamin D, important for maintaining strong, healthy bones in combination with calcium. The fat-soluble vitamin helps keep muscles strong, supports immune functions, and acts as an antioxidant to reduce the free radicals produced during exercise.

The UK Department of Health guidelines state that we should eat oily fish or another source of omega-3 at least once a week.

EAT LIKE AN ELITE

Deena Kastor's Pickled Veggie Sandwich

Winning the Olympic bronze medal for the Marathon at Athens in 2004 was the pinnacle of Deena Kastor's career. She is a three-time Olympian, won the Chicago Marathon in 2005, and still holds the US Women's Marathon record. An avid baker, writer and coach, Deena still competes as a master's runner. Her book, *Let Your Mind Run*, talks about the importance of mental strength when it comes to training.

SERVES 1

For the pickles:
150g (5½oz/1 cup) finely sliced vegetables (red onions, carrots, cauliflower or cucumber)
120ml (4fl oz/½ cup) apple cider vinegar
120ml (4fl oz/½ cup) white distilled vinegar
1 heaped Tbsp brown sugar (or honey or maple syrup)
2 heaped tsp salt (I like Maldon sea salt flakes)

To serve (per sandwich):
2 slices sourdough or wholemeal bread
your choice of protein: sliced chicken, beef or hummus (about 100g/3½oz)
thinly sliced raw beetroot (beets) (about 30g/1oz)
sliced cucumber or carrot (about 30g/1oz)
¼ avocado, peeled, pitted and sliced
sunflower seeds, for sprinkling
1 x serving of pickles (above)

Pack the sliced vegetables into an airtight container or jar.

In a small bowl, whisk together the other ingredients until the sugar has dissolved.

Pour the pickling liquid over the vegetables, seal, then shake to combine. Set aside for 10 minutes, shaking from time to time. This will make more pickles than you need, but they store well in the refrigerator for up to a week.

Build your sandwich with two slices of good bread, add your choice of protein, then stuff it full of the fresh vegetables. Finish with a sprinkling of sunflower seeds and some of the pickles.

DEENA SAYS:

'I always like a combo of carbs and protein. A sandwich or smoothie is an easy way to bring something to practice sessions, so I can eat quickly to replenish and begin rebuilding. If I'm lazy or having a busy morning, I'll bring sprouted raw almonds and an apple, but more often it's thoughtful and put together. And never the same things, because I believe in mixing up nutrients.'

Baobab Corn

Baobab is a fruit from the baobab tree – the same trees that lined the route of the Malawi Impact Marathon that I ran in 2018. Packed with vitamin C, one tablespoon of powdered baobab provides half of the recommended daily intake (RDI) for adults. Adding a spoonful of baobab powder to smoothies or yoghurt gives a sweet and tangy flavour, it is also a great way to bump up your vitamin C levels, especially during the winter months, although this recipe is more of a summer barbecue recipe. If you don't have any baobab powder to hand, it tastes just as good without!

SERVES 4

4 corn-on-the-cob (ears of corn)
60g (2¼oz/¼ cup) salted butter, melted
½ tsp cayenne pepper
1 Tbsp baobab powder, plus extra to garnish
2 limes: juice and finely grated zest of 1 lime; 1 cut into wedges to garnish
1 sprig fresh rosemary, finely chopped
salt, to taste

Preheat a large griddle pan or barbecue (outdoor grill).

Bring a large pan of salted water to the boil, add the corn and cook for 5–6 minutes until tender, then remove and set aside.

Meanwhile, mix together the butter, cayenne pepper, baobab powder, lime juice and zest, and most of the chopped rosemary.

Brush the corn with the baobab butter and griddle or barbecue for 10 minutes, turning frequently, until golden brown all over.

Brush again with the butter before serving with the remaining rosemary, a pinch of salt, a sprinkling of extra baobab powder and lime wedges on the side.

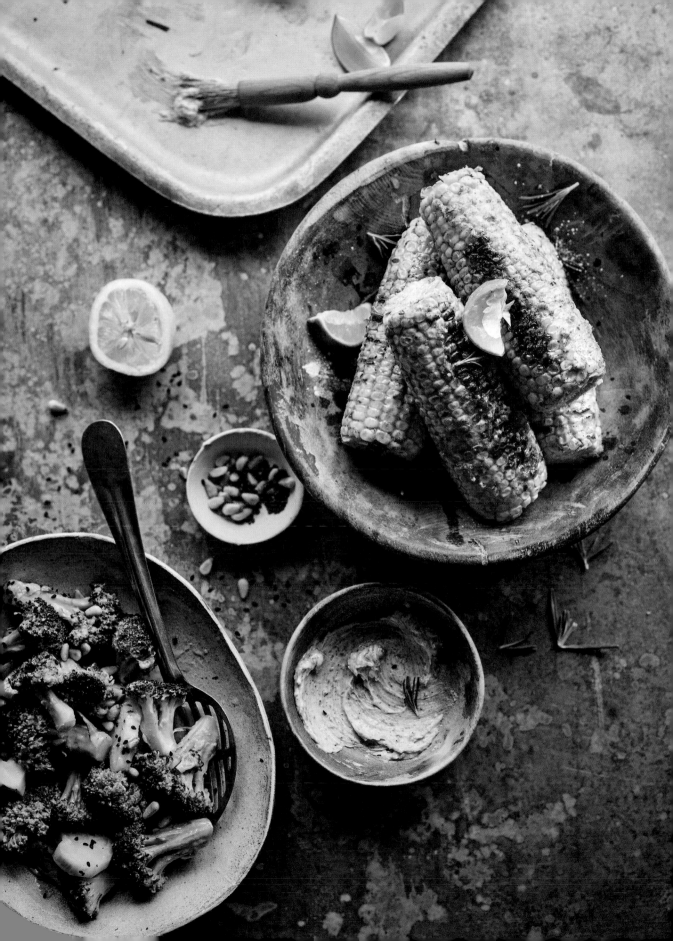

Thai Veggie Curry Soup

I learned from my Malaysian aunt that for an authentic curry, you should heat the coconut milk first, then add the paste. This is her delicious curry paste recipe, against which I now compare every other Thai green curry. Hopefully, you'll think it's as great as I do!

SERVES 4

For the curry paste:
2 spring onions (scallions), roughly chopped
1 lemongrass stalk, roughly chopped
1–2 green chillies (to taste), deseeded and roughly chopped
2 cloves garlic, roughly chopped
2.5-cm (1-in) piece fresh root ginger, peeled and roughly chopped
2 dried kaffir lime leaves
2 Tbsp reduced-salt soy sauce
1½ tsp fish sauce (optional)
large handful fresh coriander (cilantro), leaves and stalks, roughly chopped

For the soup:
1 x 400-ml (14-fl oz) can coconut milk
500ml (17fl oz/generous 2 cups) reduced-salt chicken or vegetable stock (bouillon)
1 red (bell) pepper, deseeded and finely sliced
170g (6oz) baby sweetcorn (baby corn), halved
200g (7oz) pak choi (bok choy), roughly chopped
200g (7oz) sugar snap peas, roughly chopped
200g (7oz) dried rice noodles
lime wedges, to serve

Start by making the curry paste: in a food processor, blitz together all of the paste ingredients, reserving some of the fresh coriander (cilantro) leaves to garnish.

To make the soup, bring the coconut milk and stock (bouillon) to the boil in a large saucepan. Stir through the curry paste, then add the red (bell) pepper and baby sweetcorn (baby corn). Reduce the heat and simmer for 5 minutes.

Add the pak choi (bok choy), sugar snap peas and noodles to the pan and cook for a further 3 minutes.

Divide the soup among 4 bowls and serve garnished with the lime wedges and reserved coriander leaves.

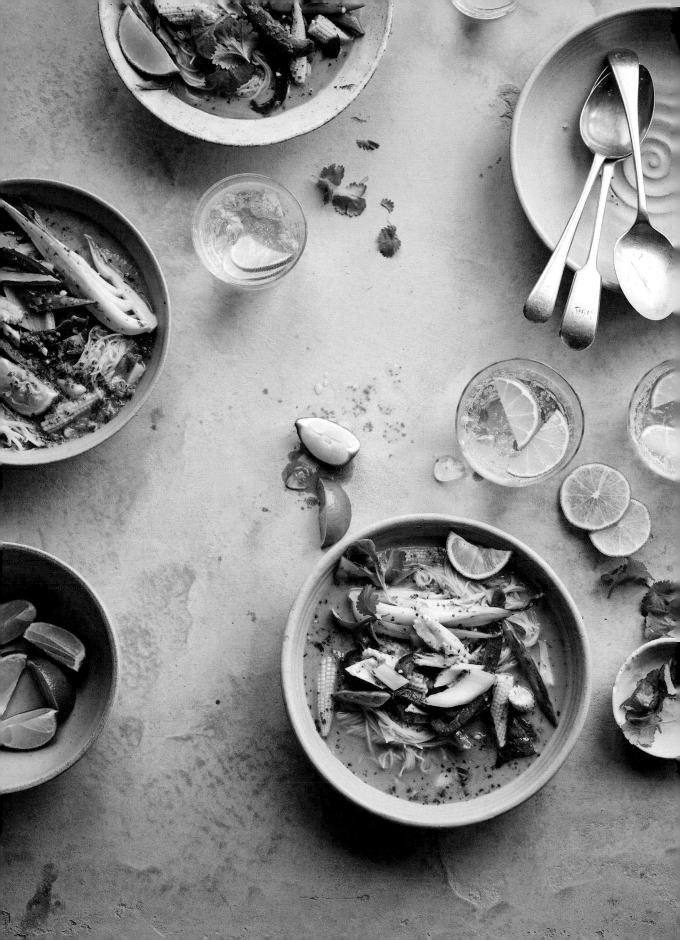

Curry-Roasted Chicken with Carrots and Gravy

There's nothing better than a homemade Sunday roast; however I often can't be bothered to make one with 'all the trimmings' after a 20-miler. This version is cooked all-in-one, with no need to peel and chop enough veg to feed an army (or hungry runners for that matter!). This works well served with the Turmeric Coconut Potatoes (see page 145).

SERVES 4 GENEROUSLY

2 limes: 1 halved; 1 cut into wedges
1 x 1.8-kg (4-lb) whole chicken
30g (1oz/2 Tbsp) butter, softened
2 Tbsp curry powder
1 clove garlic, crushed
2.5-cm (1-in) piece fresh root ginger, finely grated
½ tsp ground cumin
1 tsp ground coriander
500g (1lb 2oz) baby carrots (such as Chanteney), cleaned
¾ Tbsp plain (all-purpose) flour
1 x 165-ml (5½-fl oz) can full-fat coconut milk
150ml (5fl oz/⅔ cup) lukewarm water
salt and freshly ground black pepper, to taste
extra seasonal vegetables, to serve
mango chutney, to serve

Preheat oven to 190°C/375°F/gas mark 5.

Put the lime halves into the cavity of the chicken, tie the legs together with kitchen string and put the chicken into a large, high-sided roasting pan.

In a small bowl, mix together the softened butter, curry powder, garlic, ginger, ground cumin and coriander and some seasoning. Spread the spiced butter over the top and sides of the bird, then cover with foil and roast for 1 hour.

After 1 hour, remove the foil and add the carrots to the roasting pan, turning to coat them in the buttery juices. Return to the oven to roast for a further 20 minutes or until the carrots are tender and the chicken is cooked through (the juices should run clear when the thickest part of the leg is pierced with a knife).

Transfer the chicken to a board, cover it with foil and let rest. Spoon the carrots into a serving dish and keep warm while you make the gravy.

Spoon off and discard as much of the fat from the roasting pan as you can, leaving the cooking juices behind, then set the pan over a medium heat. Stirring continuously, add the flour, then add the coconut milk and water to the pan. Bring to a simmer and, continuing to stir, allow the gravy to thicken for 3–5 minutes. Check the seasoning and adjust to taste.

Serve the chicken, carrots and gravy with some seasonal vegetables if you like, with the lime wedges and some mango chutney on the side.

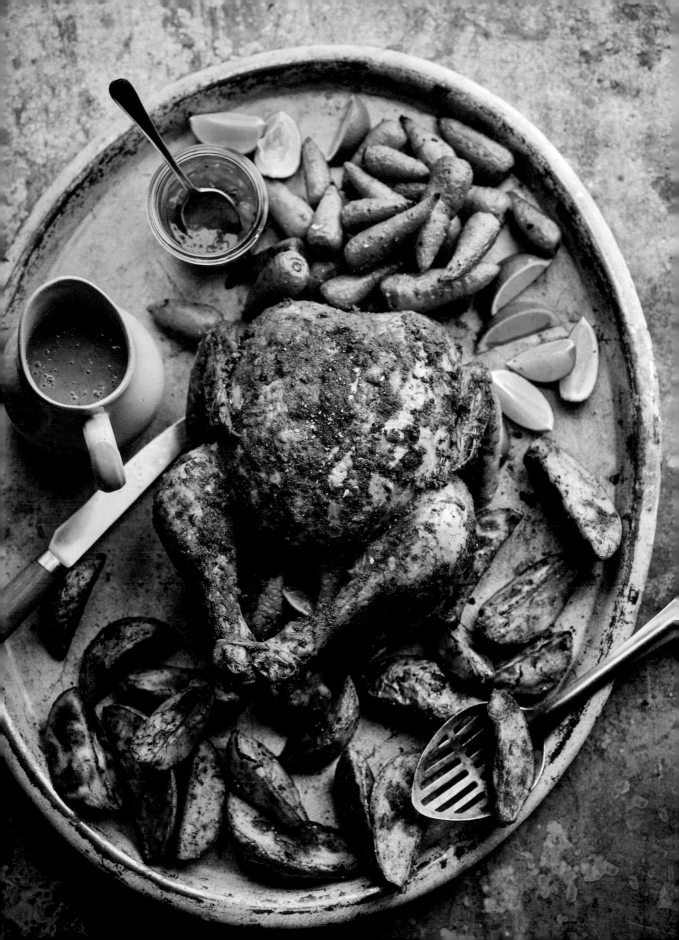

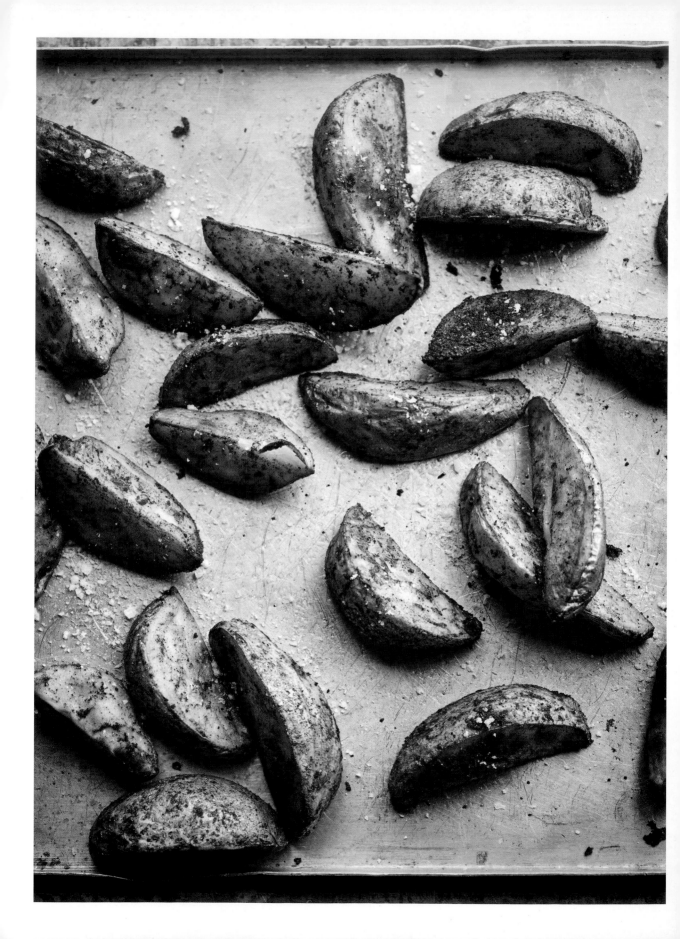

Turmeric Coconut Potatoes

With a mixture of carbs, fat and salt, these potatoes are the ultimate multi-taskers. I like to make a big batch to serve alongside roast chicken or burgers, and refrigerate some to eat on the run later. They are perfect for those who prefer something savoury for their long runs or rides, and they survive surprisingly well, even when squished in a pocket.

SERVES 4

500g (1lb 2oz) potatoes, washed
1 tsp ground turmeric
½ tsp ground cinnamon
½ tsp ground cumin
½ tsp ground coriander
1 Tbsp coconut oil
salt and ground black pepper, to taste

Preheat the oven to 200°C/400°F/gas mark 6.

Halve the potatoes, then cut each half into wedges. Transfer the potato wedges to a large bowl and toss in the spices and plenty of seasoning until evenly coated.

Meanwhile, put the coconut oil into a large roasting pan and place in the oven to melt. When melted, carefully toss the wedges through the oil in the pan until well coated, and arrange in a single layer.

Roast for 25 minutes, or until the wedges are crispy on the outside and soft inside.

Burger Bowl

These burger bowls are inspired by an amazing one I had, with running friends Heather, Kindal and Mel, in Arizona after the Phoenix-Mesa Half Marathon. It felt like the perfect mix of carbs and protein for refuelling, plus veggies to balance out our post-race frozen yoghurt with all the toppings. Similarly, if you want to use a readymade burger (be it veggie, chicken or even Lauren Fleshman's Favourite Loaded Burger, see page 148), then go for it!

SERVES 4

For the burgers:
500g (1lb 2oz) high-quality minced (ground) steak
1 small onion, finely chopped
1 medium egg
100g (3½oz/1¾ cups) fresh breadcrumbs
1 tsp Dijon mustard
salt and freshly ground black pepper, to taste

For the bowls:
2 sweet potatoes, chopped into 2.5-cm (1-in) cubes
1 red (bell) pepper, deseeded and chopped
2 Tbsp olive oil
350g (12½oz) Brussels sprouts, trimmed and halved
1 Tbsp maple syrup
1 chicken or vegetable stock (bouillon) cube
250g (9oz/1½ cups) quinoa
1 clove garlic, crushed
200g (7oz) chestnut (cremini) mushrooms, finely sliced
1 ripe avocado, peeled and sliced
ketchup, aioli or hummus, to serve

Preheat the oven to 200°C/400°F/gas mark 6.

Put the burger meat into a large mixing bowl, add the onion, egg, breadcrumbs, mustard and plenty of seasoning and mix until well combined. Divide the mixture into 4 equal pieces and shape each into a patty.

Arrange the sweet potato and red (bell) pepper in a single layer in a roasting pan, drizzle with ½ tablespoon of the oil, season well and toss to coat. Roast for 10 minutes.

Meanwhile, in a bowl, toss together the Brussels sprouts in a bowl with another ½ tablespoon of the oil, the maple syrup and plenty of seasoning. When the potatoes and peppers have had 10 minutes, remove the pan from the oven, add the sprouts and return to the oven for another 20 minutes.

Bring a large saucepan of water to the boil, add the stock (bouillon) cube and the quinoa and simmer for 15 minutes or until softened.

Meanwhile, heat the remaining 1 tablespoon oil in a large frying pan (skillet) over a medium-high heat, add the burger patties and fry for 8 minutes, turning once, until each side is well browned. Carefully transfer the burgers to a baking sheet and cook in the oven for a further 12 minutes, or until well heated through.

Return the frying pan to the heat, add the garlic and fry for 1 minute. Add the mushrooms and fry for a further 10 minutes or until golden and soft.

Build your burger bowl with a combination of quinoa, roasted veggies, fried mushrooms, sliced avocado and burgers. Serve with ketchup, aioli or hummus.

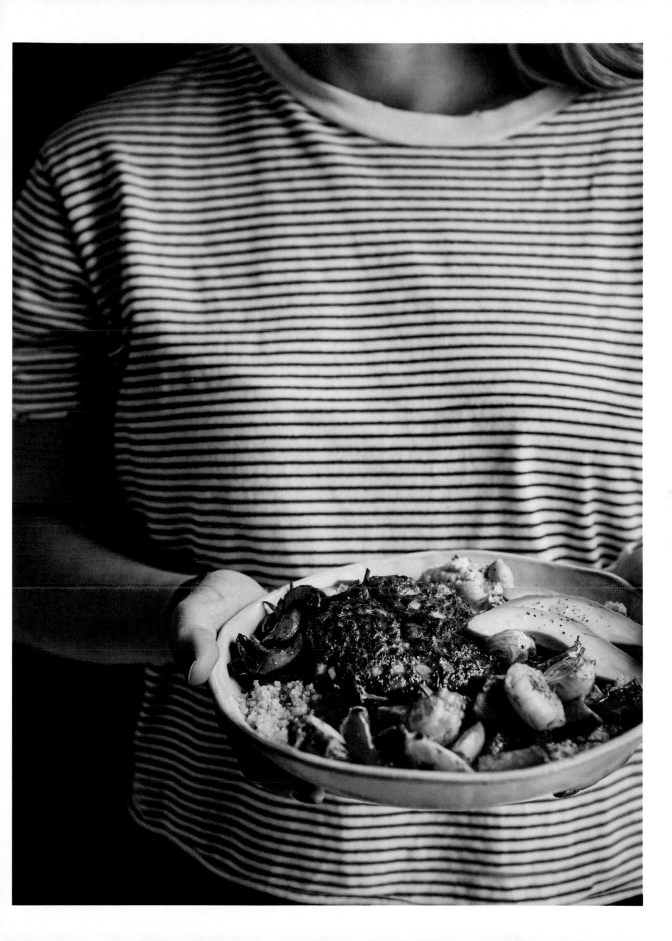

Lauren Fleshman's Favourite Loaded Burger

Lauren Fleshman is a two-time US 5000m Outdoor Track and Field Champion, and has represented the US at the World Championships three times. She made her marathon debut at the New York City Marathon in 2011, placing twelfth. She is now a Oiselle pro-runner and co-founded Picky Bars with her husband, the professional triathlete Jesse Thomas.

Make your burger extra-special by adding blue cheese to your beef patty, Lauren Fleshman-style! Alternatively, serve with a summer salad, such as the Strawberry and Halloumi Salad on page 75, subbing the halloumi for goat's cheese, adding walnuts and serving with a 'frosty stout' to be a true 'Fleshman Flyer'!

SERVES 1

1 homemade burger (see page 146) or good-quality pre-made burger
1 sourdough bun
30g (1oz) blue cheese, such as Gorgonzola or Roquefort
½ ripe avocado, peeled
handful of rocket (arugula)
1 tomato, sliced

Make and cook your burger according to the instructions on page 146, or according to the packet instructions.

Split the sourdough bun and place the cooked burger inside. Pile the blue cheese on top. Slice the avocado and place on top of the cheese, along with a handful of rocket (arugula) and a couple of slices of tomato. Serve and enjoy!

Hummus Buddha Bowl

I think that this easy dinner works at any time of the year: just swap any of the veggies for whatever is in season. This also makes a brilliant packed lunch to refuel after a midday workout, or to prepare for an evening session.

SERVES 4

1 small head cauliflower
500g (1lb 2oz) butternut
  squash, peeled and cut
  into 2.5-cm (1-in) cubes
2 Tbsp olive oil, plus extra
  if needed
1 tsp ground turmeric
½ tsp ground cumin
2 tsp paprika
1 vegetable stock (bouillon)
  cube
250g (9oz/1¼ cups) farro
  (wheat berries)
1 large courgette (zucchini),
  roughly chopped
2 (bell) peppers, deseeded
  and roughly chopped
1 x 400-g (14-oz) can
  chickpeas (garbanzo
  beans), drained and rinsed
3 Tbsp hummus
2 Tbsp full-fat natural (plain)
  or Greek yoghurt or
  dairy-free alternative
70g (2½oz/½ cup)
  pomegranate seeds
3 Tbsp pumpkin seeds
large handful rocket (arugula)
salt and freshly ground black
  pepper, to taste
2 wholemeal pita breads,
  toasted, to serve

Preheat the oven to 180°C/350°F/gas mark 4. Line a large roasting pan with baking paper.

Cut the cauliflower into small florets. Toss the florets and butternut squash together with 1½ tablespoons of the oil, the ground turmeric and cumin, and 1 teaspoon of the paprika. Spread the mixture over the roasting pan, season with salt and pepper and roast for 10 minutes.

Meanwhile, bring a large pan of water to the boil and add the stock (bouillon) cube and farro (wheat berries). Reduce to a simmer and cook for 20–25 minutes until tender. Drain and set aside.

Add the courgette (zucchini) and (bell) peppers to the cauliflower in the roasting pan and toss together, adding a little more oil if it looks dry. Roast for a further 10–15 minutes, or until the vegetables are golden and tender.

On a separate baking sheet, lay out the chickpeas (garbanzo beans) in a single layer and toss together with the remaining ½ tablespoon of oil and 1 teaspoon of paprika, and plenty of salt and pepper. Roast for 10 minutes or until slightly crispy.

In a small bowl, mix the hummus with the yoghurt and season with salt and pepper.

Put the farro into a large bowl and stir in the chickpeas. Layer the roasted vegetables on top, sprinkle over the pomegranate and pumpkin seeds and scatter over some rocket (arugula). Drizzle over most of the hummus dressing and serve with pita bread and the remaining hummus dressing on the side.

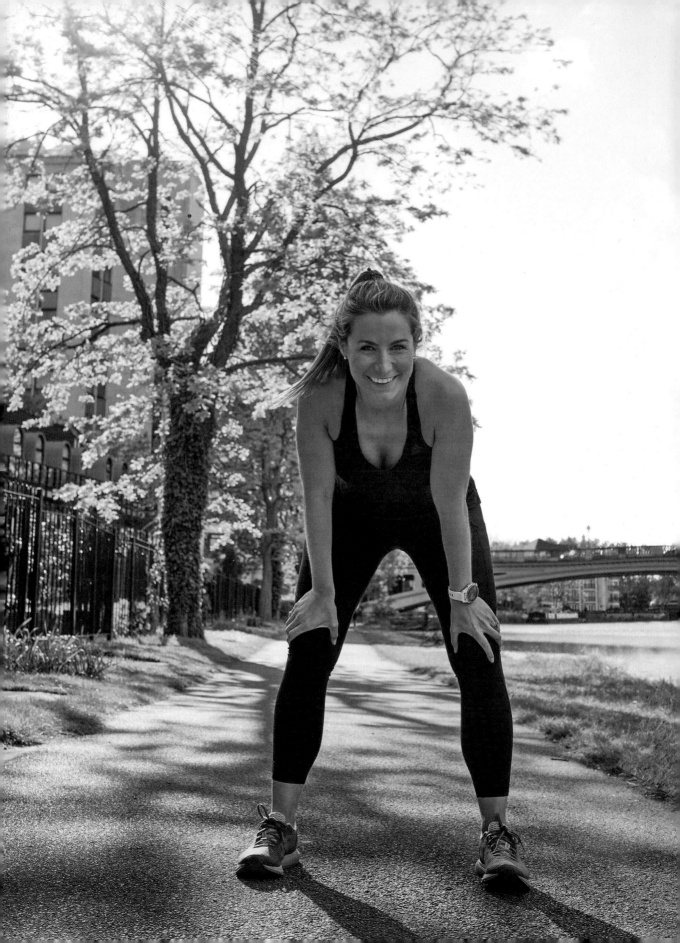

SNACKS

Elevenses are a very real thing in my life. When people say they go from breakfast to lunch without getting hungry, I am immediately suspicious of them. Maybe they don't run 8 miles before work, maybe they don't talk about food all day (job hazard of a student dietitian), or maybe their morning cereal really does tide them over. But for me, regardless of what I've eaten for breakfast, I need a mid-morning snack (and a mid-afternoon one too!).

The key to a good snack is the same as with most meals: combine protein, carbs and fat to help you feel satiated. Four o'clock became affectionately known as 'choc-o-clock' in my old office, and we'd walk up seven floors to get a cup of tea and 'something chocolatey' to satisfy the craving. I am a big chocoholic, but now I try to have a chocolate snack that will actually fill me up, provide nutrients (rather than just sugar) and fuel me for an evening run-commute or workout. My favourites are the super-simple Chocolate Fruit and Nut Snacks (page 152), the decadently fudgy Choc-O'clock Sweet Potato Brownies (page 120) or a slice of Triple Chocolate Banana Bread (page 113). The Mocha Bites (page 168) are also great if you need to get through that mid-afternoon slump and pump you up for a strength session.

For those wanting something more savoury, I recommend the Peanut Butter Hummus (page 158) with crudités or pretzels, or the Egg Muffins (page 169).

I used to struggle with what snacks to buy when I was at work, so while these aren't all recipes, I thought it would be helpful to share some ideas for things to nibble on, to keep marathon 'hanger' at bay:

- Fruit and Greek yoghurt
- Popcorn
- Trail Mix (create your own from the options on pages 164–7)
- Banana with nut butter
- Flapjacks (try the Nutty Molasses Flapjacks on page 160)
- Energy bars (try the Oat Berry Breakfast Bars on page 59)
- Milky coffee/chocolate milk (make your own, page 110)
- Piece of toast with nut butter or some avocado
- Cottage cheese
- Avocado Loaf (page 114, try the sweet version topped with some light cream cheese or nut butter)
- Homemade fruit smoothie with milk or yoghurt (for added fat/protein)

Chocolate Fruit and Nut Snacks

These make the best post-dinner evening treat or mid-afternoon pick-me-up. You can use whatever fruit or nut combination you like best, but this combination works well in the refrigerator or freezer. Two Brazil nuts a day provide your daily recommended dose of selenium. The antioxidants in selenium can help ease post-exercise cell damage, maintain thyroid function and regulate metabolism

MAKES 4 PORTIONS

30g (1oz/1 square) dark (plain unsweetened) chocolate, roughly chopped, or dairy-free alternative
2 satsumas
1 banana
12 Brazil nuts

Put the chocolate into a heatproof bowl set over a pan of gently simmering water (being careful not to let the base of the bowl touch the water). Gently stir until the chocolate has melted.

Meanwhile, peel and separate the satsuma segments, and peel and roughly chop the banana.

Line a large baking sheet with baking paper. Spread the fruit and nuts in a single layer on the sheet, then drizzle over the melted chocolate. Alternatively, half dip each piece into the chocolate and set it back on the sheet.

Chill in the refrigerator or freezer. I like to put half in the fridge for immediate consumption and leave the rest in the freezer for later in the week. Once frozen, the nuts are fine to transfer to the refrigerator, but the fruit needs to be eaten from frozen.

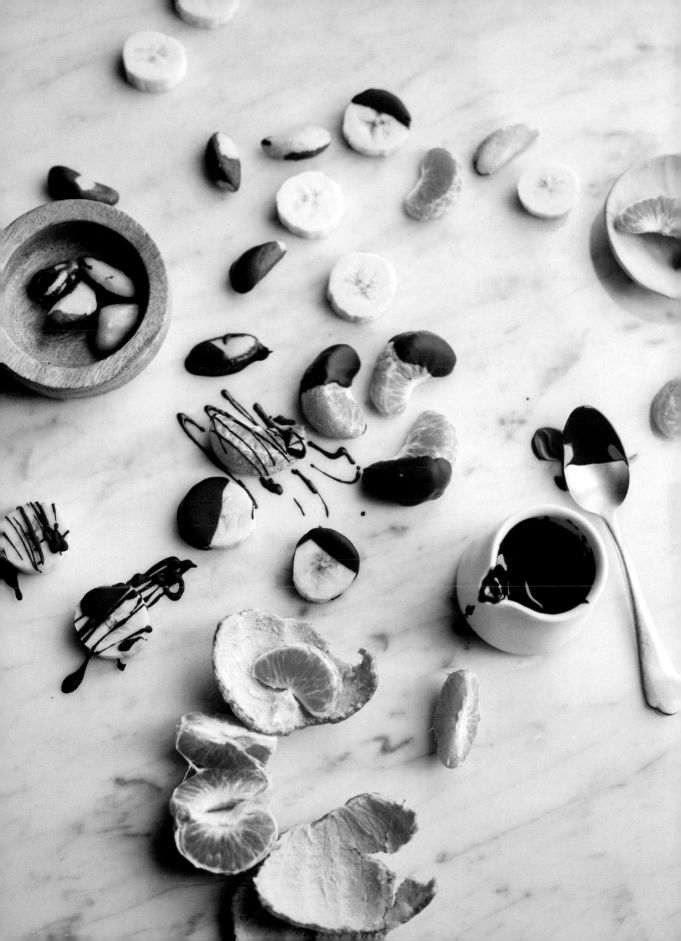

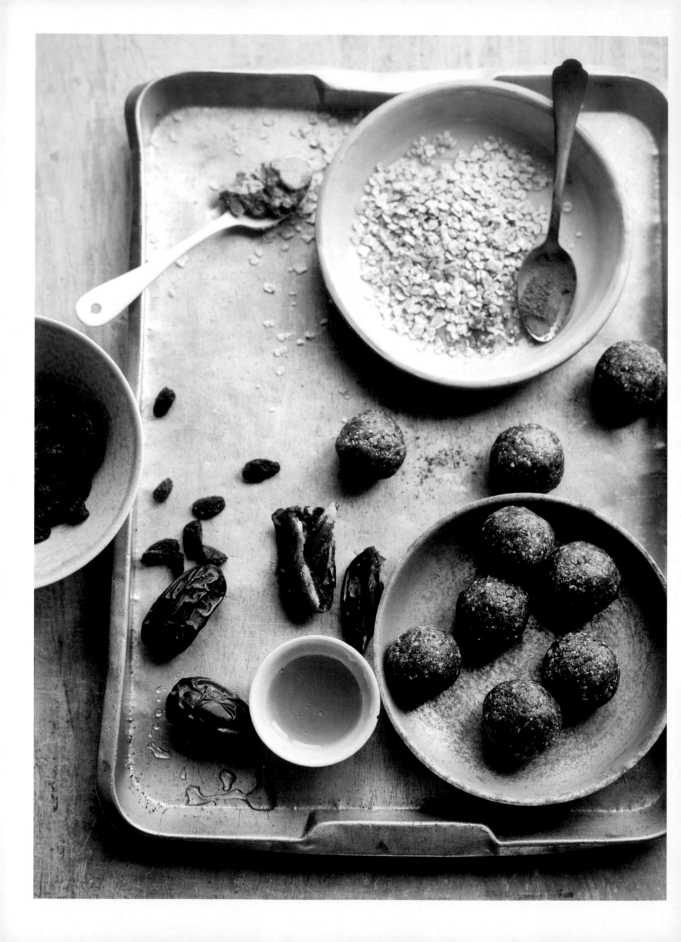

Oatmeal Raisin 'Cookies'

These were the first energy balls I ever made, years ago when they were becoming trendy. I've since made these regularly, and have a constant stash in the freezer, ready to grab and go. These also make for delicious running or cycling fuel. Leave them to defrost slightly before eating, or pack into a zip-lock bag or Tupperware container to take out with you and enjoy when fully thawed.

MAKES 20 BALLS

150g (5½oz/1½ cups) quick-cook porridge oats (instant oatmeal) or rolled (old-fashioned) oats
100g (3½oz) dates
125g (4½oz/generous ½ cup) peanut butter (smooth or chunky)
1 Tbsp ground cinnamon
1 tsp vanilla extract
1 Tbsp honey (Manuka is great for its antibacterial properties)
125g (4½oz/scant 1 cup) raisins or sultanas (golden raisins)

Put the oats into a food processor and pulse for 20 seconds if using quick-cook oats (oatmeal) or 1 minute if using rolled (old-fashioned) oats. Add the dates, peanut butter, cinnamon, vanilla and honey, and pulse for about 1 minute, until the mixture starts to come together. Add the raisins and pulse for another 15 seconds.

Line a baking sheet with baking paper. Divide the mixture into 20 small balls (each about the size of a walnut). You may need to really squeeze them to bring them together. Arrange on the baking tray and chill or freeze until solid.

Beetroot Cacao Coconut Balls

Beetroot (beets) is one of the best superfoods for runners – see below for all the reasons why. Rolling these beetroot cacao balls in coconut prevents that tell-tale, bright red fingertip staining that will give away any secret afternoon snacking. They can get a bit squishy when it's warm, so keep them in a ziplock bag or sealed container in a pocket or bag if you want to enjoy them on the run.

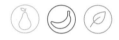

MAKES 16

1 cooked beetroot (beet),
    roughly chopped
5 Medjool dates
1 Tbsp cacao powder
30g (1oz/⅓ cup) pecans,
    roughly chopped
50g (2oz/½ cup) ground
    almonds
30g (1oz/generous ⅓ cup)
    desiccated (dried shredded)
    coconut, plus extra to
    decorate
1 vanilla pod, seeds scraped

In a food processor, blitz together the beetroot (beet), dates, cacao powder and pecans. Add the almonds, coconut and vanilla seeds and pulse until combined.

Line a baking sheet with baking paper. Place the extra coconut in a shallow bowl.

Roll the mixture into 16 small balls (each about the size of a walnut), then roll in the coconut until covered. Lay on the baking sheet and freeze for 1–2 hours until solid.

Transfer to an airtight container and store in the refrigerator for up to 1 week, or in the freezer for up to 1 month.

SUPERFOOD BEETROOT

Ever seen anyone drink a bottle of concentrated beetroot (beet) juice pre-race? Well, studies have shown that consuming beetroot before a race can decrease your time over 5K, and improve cardio-respiratory endurance in athletes, therefore increase performance and extending time to exhaustion.

The magic in the beetroot comes from the nitrates (also found in dark leafy greens). Nitrates are converted into nitric oxide in the body, which helps increase blood flow to the muscles, encourages mitochondrial growth and strengthens muscle contractions, enhancing athlete endurance (one study even suggests by as much as 16 per cent).

Ginger and Molasses Energy Bars

Here's a snack you can eat the on-the-run without the need for an aid-station set up, or just at your desk while dreaming of the trails.

MAKES 24 SQUARES

50g (2oz/½ cup) jumbo (old-fashioned) oats
200g (7oz/1½ cups) plain (all-purpose) flour, sifted
¼ tsp ground cloves
1 tsp ground ginger
1 tsp ground cinnamon
1 tsp bicarbonate of soda (baking soda)
120ml (4fl oz/½ cup) vegetable oil (or other unflavoured oil – I use avocado)
50g (2oz/2½ Tbsp) molasses or treacle
150g (5½oz/¾ cup) light brown sugar
1 large egg, beaten
2 Tbsp finely chopped crystallized (candied) ginger

Preheat the oven to 180°C/350°F/gas mark 4. Grease and line a 20-cm (8-in) square baking tin (pan) with baking paper.

In a large bowl, mix together the oats, flour, spices and bicarbonate of soda (baking soda).

In a separate bowl, whisk together the oil, molasses or treacle, sugar and egg.

Pour the wet ingredients into the dry and stir to combine; the mixture will be quite thick. Spoon the mixture into the prepared tin and press down, making sure it reaches into the corners (this might be easiest with your hands). Sprinkle over the crystallized (candied) ginger.

Bake for 20–25 minutes until the top is golden and crisp, and the middle is just set.

Leave to cool in the tin, then cut into 24 squares. These last for up to 5 days in an airtight container.

Peanut Butter Hummus

I can't remember when hummus became a staple in my refrigerator, but it has definitely been on my weekly shopping list for years now. At any given time, I have at least three different flavour selections in stock – usually a combination of homemade and store-bought options. It's a great serving of protein to keep you full for longer and, served with crudités, makes the perfect mid-morning, afternoon or evening snack. I try to have carrot sticks and a pot of hummus on hand to snack on while I prepare dinner, to avoid opening a bag of crisps (chips) and to help me get in an extra serving of veg.

I first tried peanut butter hummus at a Peruvian restaurant in London last year and couldn't believe I hadn't made it before.

MAKES 8–12 SERVINGS (DEPENDING ON POST-RUN HUNGER)

1 x 400-g (14-oz) can chickpeas (garbanzo beans)
1 small clove garlic, crushed
4 Tbsp smooth or crunchy peanut butter
juice of ½–1 lemon (according to taste)
¼ tsp ground cumin
1 tsp tahini
2 Tbsp olive oil
salt and freshly ground black pepper, to taste
crudités (such as carrot, cucumber or celery sticks) or crackers, to serve

In a large food processor, blitz together the chickpeas (garbanzo beans), garlic, peanut butter, lemon juice, ground cumin, tahini and olive oil, until well combined. With the motor running, slowly add 3 tablespoons water, blending until fully combined and the mixture reaches a spreadable consistency. Add a little more water if you'd like a thinner hummus. Season to taste.

Serve with your choice of crudités for dipping or with crackers for spreading.

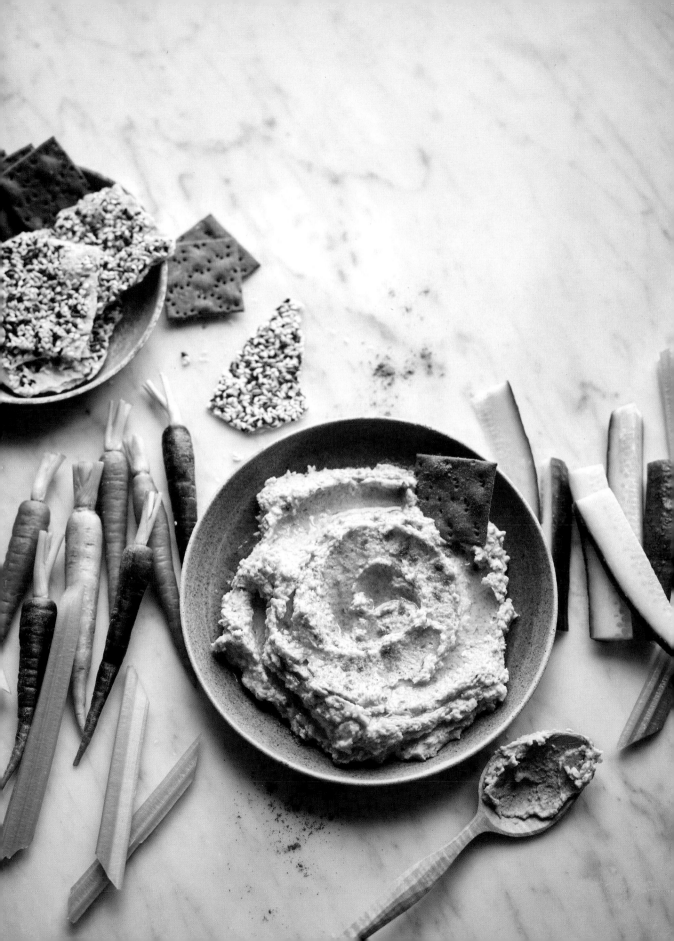

Nutty Molasses Flapjacks

Nothing says 'amateur endurance athlete' more than a flapjack (in my opinion). They are a staple at the end of many races and at Ultrarun aid stations. Perfect for on the run, or with a cup of tea pre- or post-run.

MAKES 16

250g (9oz/2½ cups) jumbo (old-fashioned) oats
50g (2oz/½ cup) pecans, roughly chopped
50g (2oz/scant ½ cup) Brazil nuts, roughly chopped
80g (3oz/⅓ cup) unsalted butter
120g (4½oz/6 Tbsp) golden syrup
80g (3oz/4 Tbsp) molasses or treacle
1 tsp ground ginger

Preheat the oven to 180°C/350°F/gas mark 4. Line a 20-cm (8-in) square baking tin (pan) and a large baking sheet with baking paper.

Spread the oats and nuts over the baking sheet and toast in the oven for 10 minutes.

Meanwhile, in a large saucepan over a low heat, gently melt together the butter, golden syrup, molasses or treacle and ground ginger, stirring regularly so that the mixture doesn't stick.

Pour the toasted oats and nuts into the molasses mixture and stir to combine, making sure that all the oats are evenly coated. Spoon into the prepared tin and press together, levelling the top. Bake for 25 minutes.

Leave to cool in the tin, then cut into 16 squares and store in an airtight container.

SUPERFOOD: MOLASSES

Thick, syrupy molasses – also known as black treacle – is a by-product of the sugar-refining process. Its vitamin and mineral content is higher than regular sugar and it is packed with iron, calcium, potassium and magnesium, making it the perfect addition to your repertoire of on-the-run sweet treat recipes.

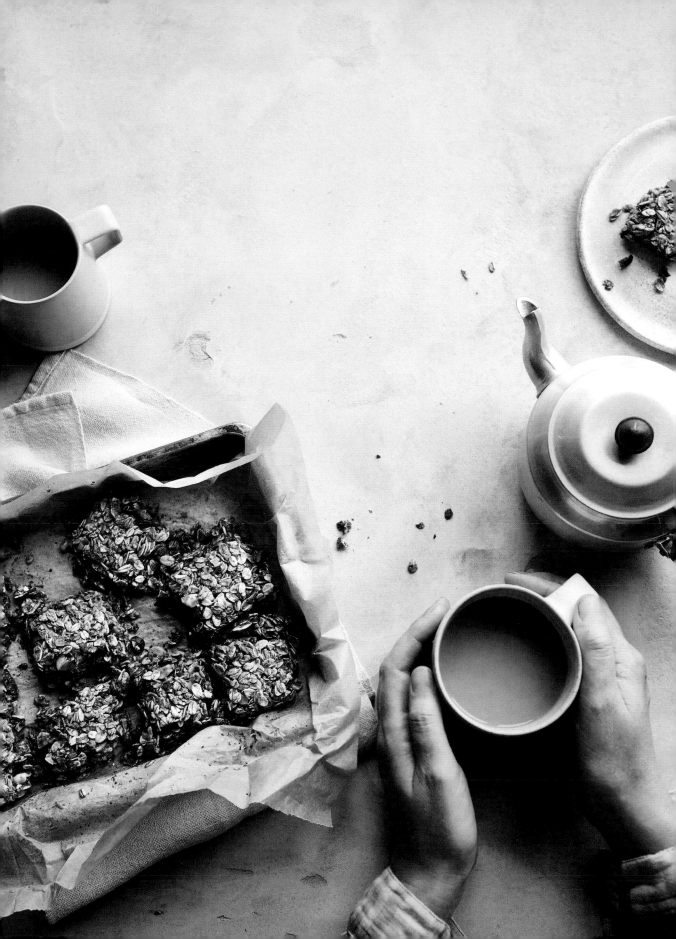

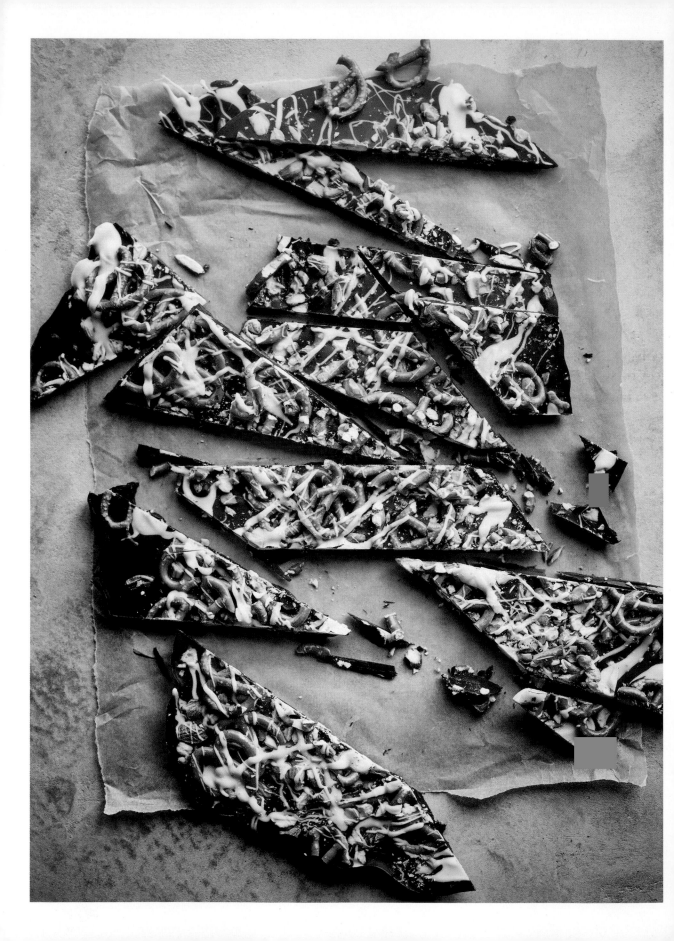

Pretzel Bark

Chocolate-covered pretzels are one of my all-time favourite snacks and I try to limit myself to only buying them in the airport as a treat. However, as I find myself flying more and more to the US for work trips, that trick isn't working so well.

Confession: After a half marathon, I once drove 20 minutes in the wrong direction from my house, just to buy chocolate-covered pretzels. And I ate them all in the car on the drive back...

So, with all that in mind, I wanted to create a recipe that satisfied the sweet-salty craving, but that wouldn't have you (okay, me) reaching the bottom of the bag before you've made it home. Using dark chocolate reduces the sugar content, but still provides that delicious chocolate taste, while the pretzels and pistachios should keep you satiated for longer. The white chocolate adds a little sweetness back in, but is mainly here because it looks pretty.

Feel free to use whichever nuts, dried fruit, pretzel sticks, etc. that you have at home. I also think adding dried cranberries to this would make a pretty and thoughtful homemade Christmas present!

MAKES 10 SERVINGS

400g (14oz/scant 3 cups) dark (plain unsweetened) chocolate, finely chopped
100g (3½oz/1 cup) shelled pistachios, roughly chopped
50g (2oz/1 cup) salted pretzels, lightly crushed
50g (2oz/scant ½ cup) white chocolate, finely chopped

Melt the chopped dark (plain) chocolate in a bain marie or a heatproof bowl set over a pan of barely simmering water, ensuring the base of the bowl does not touch the water.

Line a deep baking tray (lipped baking sheet), about 25 x 28cm (10 x 11in), with baking paper. Pour in the melted chocolate and spread into a thick, even layer. Working quickly while the chocolate is still liquid, sprinkle the pistachios and pretzels evenly over the chocolate.

Melt the chopped white chocolate using the same method as before. Once melted, drizzle it over the surface of the dark chocolate bark.

Chill in the refrigerator for 20 minutes or until set, then cut into large shards. Store in an airtight container in a cool, dark place or in the refrigerator if it's very hot or if you prefer chocolate cold.

Trail Mix

When creating a trail mix, or any snack, you're looking to get a balance of protein, carbohydrates and fat, to help keep you full for longer.
A good portion size is 30–40g/1–1½oz (around 150–200 calories). Try to include a rough ratio of two parts nuts to one part seeds and one part dried fruit/extras (e.g. 20g/¾oz nuts; 10g/⅓oz seeds; 10g/⅓oz fruit).

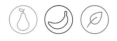

PISTACHIOS

These green beauties are rich in vitamin K and potassium, which are crucial for runners' bone health and help keep muscle tissues healthy. Potassium is a particularly key electrolyte for runners: deficiency can cause muscle weakness, fatigue and possible cramping. 100g (3½oz) of shelled pistachios will provide 29 per cent of your daily recommended intake.

ALMONDS

Raw, skin-on almonds are a great snack, either as part of a nut mix or on their own. Not only do they provide a protein punch, but you'll also benefit from the fibre, calcium, magnesium and potassium content. Studies have also shown that, when eaten with sugary items (with a high glycaemic index), almonds help reduce the overall glycaemic load of the meal.

WALNUTS

Walnuts are a great source of omega-3 fat. The body cannot manufacture these essential fatty acids, so we must include them in our diet. These fats can help reduce inflammation in the body (helpful when you have DOMS [delayed onset muscle soreness]), can help you heal faster, and are heart and brain protective.

CASHEWS

Many runners bathe in magnesium bath salts, but eating just 100g (3½oz) of cashews provides 21 per cent of our daily recommended intake of magnesium. This helps to protect the body from muscle fatigue and soreness – perfect after a hard workout. Cashews are also lower in fat than most nuts. Enjoy them raw, or soak them overnight and blitz into a cashew cream.

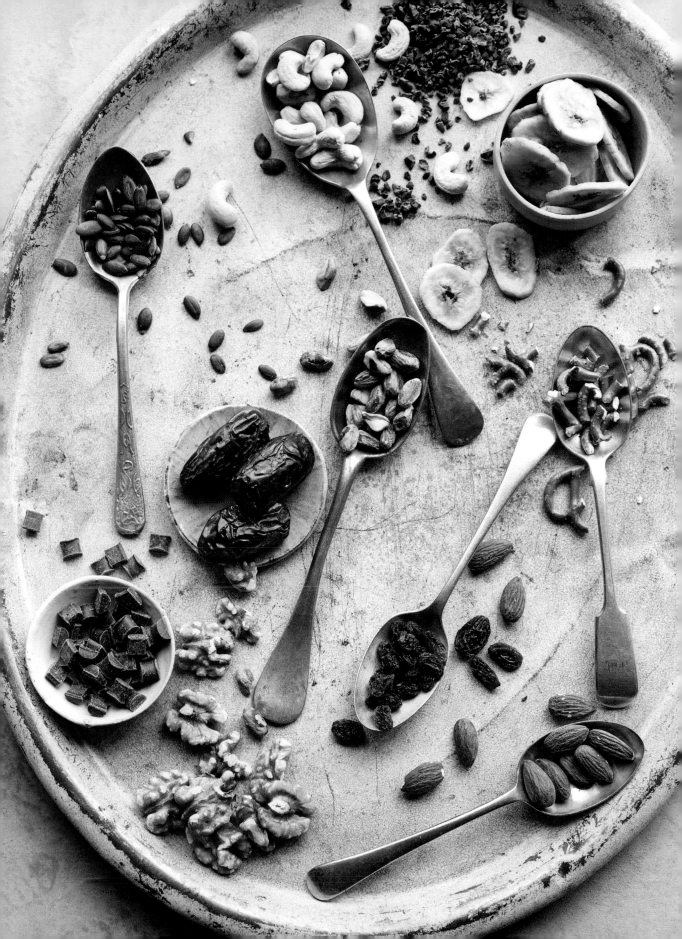

BRAZIL NUTS

Just 2 Brazil nuts provide enough selenium to meet your daily recommended intake. The human body uses selenium to produce antioxidant enzymes that can help offset damage caused by free radicals during high-intensity and endurance exercise.

MACADAMIA NUTS

Packed with thiamine, which helps your body metabolize carbohydrates into usable energy, it might be time to add these to your carb-loading plan.

HAZELNUTS

These boast the highest concentration of folate of any nuts, while also containing magnesium, calcium and potassium. Sadly, you don't get these benefits from Nutella... but chuck some dark chocolate chips into your trail mix for the best of both.

PUMPKIN SEEDS

Add these to snacks, salads or breakfasts as a source of protein, fibre and healthy fats. They're also a great source of zinc, potassium and magnesium. Zinc plays a role in our immune system function – keeping your zinc levels topped up during cold and flu season (or when you're feeling run down during marathon training) is really important.

SUNFLOWER SEEDS

A 30g (1oz) dose of these provides your recommended daily intake of vitamin E, which may prevent heart disease, as well as promoting immune system health and reducing inflammation. You'll also get a dose of selenium and copper alongside the fibre and protein boost.

CHESTNUTS

A great source of carbohydrates (perfect to fuel a workout), not to mention vitamin B, fibre, and copper – a trace mineral that is involved in bone strength and boosting the immune system.

RAISINS

These are a great natural alternative to commercial sports supplements – a study found similar performance benefits in runners using raisins as those using sports chews when compared with water alone in a 5K time trial. Not only are they cheap, but they also have naturally occurring potassium and iron, too.

DATES

Dates seem to be a superfood in their own right; they certainly are nature's candy. Just 2 Medjool dates provide 33g (1¼oz) of carbohydrates and 15 per cent of your daily recommended fibre intake (this high fibre content makes them a slow-release carb, helping you stay energized all afternoon). And with more potassium than bananas, these sweet treats can help your body regain electrolyte balance after a sweaty workout. Try the Super Stuffed Dates on page 38.

DRIED CHERRIES

You can read all about the power of cherries on page 33 (try making Molly Huddle's Tart Cherry Jelly), and while I'm not making a case for eating raw tart cherries on their own, even the dried sweeter versions can have benefits. Vitamin C, folate, iron and potassium are all vitamins and minerals found in these small berries, which will help boost your immune system. They also contain melatonin, which can aid sleep.

DRIED BANANAS

With plenty of carbs packed into a small portion, you can get a lot of bang for your buck with dried bananas. Plus, you'll get a dose of the essential electrolytes all runners need (potassium, magnesium and phosphorus) in each serving. Try to look for dried bananas without added sugar.

CACAO NIBS

Containing theobromine, a natural energy booster, plus a little caffeine boost, adding cacao nibs to your trail mix means you'll be ready for that evening run or gym session. Not only that, but a 28g (1oz) serving contains 4g (½oz) protein and 9g (⅓oz) fibre, as well as maganese, copper, magnesium, phosphorous, iron, zinc and calcium.

PECANS

Pecans are my favourite nut. They are actually one of the top 15 sources of antioxidants according to a 2004 study. They have been shown to prevent LDL ('bad') cholesterol from building up in your arteries and to lower total cholesterol. Plus, they're packed with phytosterols that might help protect against cardiovascular disease.

PRETZELS

With a combination of carbs and salt, these snacks are high in energy, easy to digest and help to restore sodium levels meaning they are a post-race goody-bag favourite for a reason. You could also try them in the Chocolate Pretzel Bark (page 163) to really improve your afternoon snack!

Mocha Bites

What goes better together than chocolate and coffee (especially when you need a mid-afternoon caffeine pick-me-up). A number of studies have shown a link between caffeine intake and exercise performance, improving run speed and allowing athletes to train with a greater power output or for longer after caffeine consumption. So team that mocha bite with a cup of tea or coffee and get ready to work out!

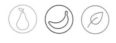

MAKES 24

200g (7oz/scant 2 cups) pecans
500g (1lb 2oz/scant 4 cups) Medjool dates, pitted
3 Tbsp desiccated (dried shredded) coconut
3 Tbsp maple syrup
1–2 Tbsp almond butter
1–2 Tbsp finely ground coffee beans or 2 tsp instant espresso powder, to taste
3 Tbsp cacao powder, or to taste, plus (optional) extra for dusting

In a food processor, pulse the pecans into small pieces. Add the dates and pulse again, then add the remaining ingredients and blitz until the mixture clumps together. Taste and add more coffee or cacao to the mix, as you prefer.

Divide the mixture equally into 24, and roll into balls, about the size of a walnut. To make them look really posh, you can also roll them in extra cacao so that they look like truffles.

Freeze or refrigerate until you want to eat them.

Egg Muffins

These make great post-run, grab-and-go breakfast items that can be eaten in the car or on the train with minimal fuss, or popped into the refrigerator at work for a mid-morning snack that will actually keep you full until lunch. Full disclosure: I need at least two if having these for breakfast!

MAKES 12

150g (5½oz) asparagus
   spears (thin ones are best),
   chopped
4 spring onions (scallions),
   finely sliced
100g (3½oz) sun-dried
   tomatoes, roughly chopped
10 large eggs
70g (2½oz) feta cheese or
   goat's cheese, crumbled
salt and freshly ground black
   pepper, to taste

Preheat the oven to 180°C/350°F/gas mark 4. Lightly grease a 12-hole muffin tin (pan) and evenly divide the chopped vegetables among the holes of the muffin tin.

In a large jug, whisk together the eggs with plenty of seasoning, then stir in the feta. Pour the egg mixture over the vegetables in the muffin tin. Bake for 12–15 minutes until the egg mixture is set.

Remove from the oven and serve warm or at room temperature. Extra muffins can be stored in the refrigerator for up to 4 days. Microwave on high for 30 seconds to reheat before serving, if you like.

Index

Acknowledgements

This book has been a labour of love. Having worked at *Good Housekeeping* writing recipes every month, I had no idea how intensive it would be to create 75+ recipes for a book.

Huge thanks goes to my husband, Tom. As he'll tell you, he wouldn't call himself a runner but he's run two marathons which I am incredibly proud of him for. He is pretty patient with my own running exploits, and very supportive of my career change into dietetics. Tom, I'm sorry I make a huge mess in the kitchen and often use every bowl, plate and saucepan. Thank you for washing up constantly while I was recipe testing (and every single night).

My Mum will be the first to admit that food and cooking isn't her thing, but I am so grateful that she taught me to cook at a young age, bought me a Jamie Oliver cookbook aged 10 and let me experiment to my heart's content in the kitchen. She was a major help in testing these recipes, going to the supermarket multiple times to get more ingredients, giving constructive feedback and generally being my number one cheerleader.

This book would not have happened without my friend and mentor, Meike Beck. She taught me pretty much everything I know about writing a recipe, thoroughly testing them and making sure they work everytime. I also learned quite a bit about the ideal gin and tonic under her tutelage. She has been a sounding board over the years for me and I couldn't have asked for a better first boss.

Thank you to my friends and family for allowing me to use their recipes in the book, for being a constant support, testing recipes for me and enthusiastically sharing others. Many of my friends and family don't run and yet have pre-ordered this book without hesitation, your excitement for all I do is not something I take for granted.

And to those new friends who I have made through running and instagram, I am so grateful that the square world brought us together. Special shout out here goes to Lindsay Hein who connected me with most of the elite runners who supplied recipes, she was so generous with her time and contacts (you should listen to her podcast 'I'll Have Another' for great running motivation, interviews with athletes and everyday runners, it's my favourite).

Gabriella, Fred, Camilla and Ulrika, thank you for being my recipe guinea pigs on countless occasions, and for giving your suggestions for which dishes should make it into the book (or not!).

Thank you must also go to my publishers at Quadrille, to Sarah, Emily and Stacey for your patience as I juggled finishing my degree and writing/editing this book. Who knew each deadline for my dissertation would match so closely with the book deadlines, hey!? And to the staff at London Met for being so flexible and supportive throughout these final months. To Maja Smend for the gorgeous photos and Pip and Libby for recreating these recipes so beautifully and reassuring me that they worked! I am so appreciative to have had such a friendly, fun yet diligent team to help make my cookbook dreams come true!

Publishing Director
Sarah Lavelle

Assistant Editor
Stacey Cleworth

Copy Editor
Emily Preece-Morrison

Consultant Dietitian
Sian Porter

Art Direction and Design
Emily Lapworth

Photographer
Maja Smend

Food Stylist
Pip Spence

Prop Stylist
Polly Webb-Wilson

Production Director
Stephen Lang

Production Controller
Sinead Hering

First published in 2019 by Quadrille,
an imprint of Hardie Grant Publishing

Quadrille
52–54 Southwark Street
London SE1 1UN
quadrille.com

Text © Charlie Watson 2019
Photography © Maja Smend 2019
Design and layout © Quadrille Publishing Limited 2019

Cataloguing in Publication Data: a catalogue record for this book is available from the British Library.

ISBN: 978 1 78713 429 4

Printed in China